PERSONAL DATA SHEET

Name _____

Address _____

Telephone _____

Birth Date _____ Height _____ Weight _____

Blood Type _____ Last Tetanus Booster Shot _____

List Allergies _____

In Case of Accident, Notify _____

Address _____

Name of Boat _____ Home Port: _____

Boat Registration Number _____

Diver Certification Agency <u>NAUI   NASDS   PADI   SSI</u>
<u>YMCA   ACUC   OTHER</u> _____

Certification Level: Diver _____

Instructor _____ Other _____

Diving Areas Commonly Used _____

_____

Boating Areas Commonly Used _____

_____

Family Physician _____

Address _____

Telephone: Home _____ Office _____

Hospital _____

Address _____

Telephone _____

ACCIDENT DATA FOR ATTENDING PHYSICIAN

NAME _____

DATE _____ Time of Day _____

Dive with Scuba _____ Dive without Scuba _____

Approximate Depth of Dive _____ Feet

Number of Dives in 12-Hour Period Preceding Accident

_____

List Any Known Disabilities of Victim _____

_____

Names of Diving Companions _____

_____

First Aid Rendered _____

_____

_____

_____

The diver's companion should accompany the victim if possible. If not, it is essential to send along the information outlined on this page.

RECOMPRESSION-CHAMBER FACILITIES

Diving Sites Most Used _____

Nearest Compression Chamber _____

Address _____

_____ Tel. _____

Distance from Most-Used Diving Sites _____ Miles

Person in Charge _____

Other Chambers in Order of Nearness

2 _____ Tel. _____

3 _____ Tel. _____

Nearest Police Facility _____ Tel. _____

Gas & Electric Tel. No. _____

Fire Rescue Service Nearest to Dive Site _____

_____ Tel. _____

Nearest Coast Guard Rescue Unit _____

Nearest Air-Sea Rescue Unit _____

_____ Tel. _____

Dial 512-LEO-FAST for Pressure-Related Emergency Information 24 hours a day.

Contents

1. General First Aid   6
   First Considerations   7
   Bleeding   8
   Shock   12
   Drowning   16
   Stoppage of Breathing   16
   Mouth-to-Mouth Resuscitation   17
   Choking and Strangulation   19
   Heart Attack   22
   Heart Failure   23
   Cardiopulmonary Resuscitation (CPR)   23
   Wound Care   26
   Broken Bones   28
   Burns   32
   Electric Shock   38
   Fainting   38
   External Ear Infection   39
   Poisoning by Mouth   39
   Poisoning by Plants   41
   Appendicitis   41
   Sprains and Strains   42
   Nosebleed   43
   Stings and Bites   44
   Snakebites   47
   Animal and Human Bites   51
   Chilling/Hypothermia   51
   Frostbite and Cold Exposure   53
   Exhaustion Syndrome   56
   Heatstroke   56
   Motion Sickness   57
   Dermatitis   57
   Ear Injuries   58
   Sore Throat   61
   Sinusitis   62
   Colds   63
   Rupture (Hernia)   63
   Stroke   64
   Toothache with Swelling   65
   Emergency Childbirth   66

2. Injuries Caused by Marine Life   70
   Marine Plants   70
   Coral   70
   Sea Urchin   71
   Cone Shells   71

Jellyfish, Sea Nettles, Portuguese Man-of-War,
   Sea Wasp   72
Octopus   72
Sting Rays   73
Venomous Fish   74
Bite Wounds   74
Sea Snakes   75
Eating Inedible Marine Animals   76

3. Pressure-Related Illness and Injury   78
   Decompression Sickness   78
   Air Embolism   79
   Mediastinal Emphysema   80
   Subcutaneous Emphysema   81
   Pneumothorax   81
   Unconscious Diver   82
   Squeeze   82
   Oxygen Shortage (Hypoxia)   83
   Oxygen Toxicity   84
   Carbon Dioxide Excess (Hypercapnia)   85
   Nitrogen Narcosis   85
   Carbon-Monoxide Poisoning   85
   Drowning   86
   Diving Above Sea Level   87
   Flying After Diving   88
   Alcohol and Marijuana   88

4. The Uses of Boating and Diving Gear for
First Aid   89
   Emergency Use of Boating Equipment   89
   Mask   89
   Snorkel   90
   Fins   91
   Wet Suit   92
   Buoyancy Compensator   92
   Knife   92
   Game Bag   96
   Spears   97

5. First-Aid Kit for Divers   98

6. First-Aid Kit for Boaters   106
   Diver First-Aid Commandments   107
   About the Council for National Cooperation
     in Aquatics   107
   Constituent Groups: CNCA and CCCA   108
   About Sea Grant   110

Index   112

1
General first aid

First aid is the immediate, emergency assistance properly given on site as soon as feasible before the victim can be placed in the hands of a professional medical practitioner. Time is important in the rendering of first aid. In the period following injury or illness, you may be the one on whom the victim totally depends. What you do may mean the difference between complete recovery and permanent disability or even death.

Diving and boating can present specialized problems that do not occur on land. Often, members of the medical profession will depend on the information you supply. Such specialized problems as depth and pressure are not commonly part of the general practitioner's service area. If not correctly identified, the symptoms of embolism, or "bends," may easily be misinterpreted and mistreated.

This handbook, designed especially for the skin and scuba diver as well as the mariner, should be carefully studied. It has been kept brief in an effort to deal with essential needs and to make it a readily portable part of your diving or boating gear. While it deals mainly with problems associated with diving, it also carries information on many problems related to surface first aid. Broken bones, bleeding, shock and poisoning are also a frequent consequence of sea accidents. This revision carries a great deal of first aid applicable to the mariner or boater. Many divers own boats or have to be ferried to special diving sites by boat, so the text was expanded to include first aid for mariners.

Most of the problems covered here are discussed in greater detail in *The New Science of Skin and Scuba Diving,* also published under the auspices of CNCA by Association Press/Follett Publishing Company. That volume should be studied thoroughly in connection with this brief manual.

FIRST CONSIDERATIONS

Three areas need to be considered promptly: a) Is the victim breathing? b) Is the victim bleeding? c) What is the cardiac condition as noted by the pulse?

Mouth-to-mouth resuscitation must be employed if the victim is not breathing. See page 17.

Severe bleeding needs to be dealt with immediately, as heavy blood loss can result in death in a few minutes. See page 9. Cardiac chest compressions may be employed if the heartbeat is not present. See page 23.

Since serious injuries are usually followed by shock, it is important to deal with this problem, which can be as serious as the injury.

An unconscious diver should be considered to have an embolism except in cases where another cause can be easily identified. In the event of a suspected embolism, the victim should be placed in a pressure chamber and pressurized to 165 feet as rapidly as possible. Necessary first aid can be given en route to the chamber and even in the chamber as required. (See Embolism, page 79.)

Moving the Victim

If back or neck injuries are involved, be careful of the method used to move the injured. See page 32. Keep patient quiet and lying down. Keep warm and try to avoid chilling. If exposed to dampness and cold, place blankets or clothing over and under the victim. Do not try to provide additional heat as this could draw the blood to the skin surface and away from the vital organs where it is needed most.

Vomiting

If victim is vomiting, turn head to one side to avoid choking.

Heat

Do not apply excessive heat as it might draw the blood from the vital organs where it is needed.

Help

Assign someone to get medical help while you apply first aid. Be sure to alert medical personnel to the details of the accident, paying special attention to depth/pressure circumstances.

BLEEDING

Bleeding in diving accidents may result from many causes; it is important to identify the probable cause and to be aware that other serious injuries may be present. Apart from bleeding caused by pressure, the victim may have suffered internal injuries that cause bleeding.

Mouth, ear, or nose bleeding suggests a pressure-type accident. Frothless blood leaking from the mouth of an unconscious diver may be the result of tongue bite made during convulsions accompanying oxygen toxicity. Frothy blood coming from the mouth of an unconscious diver suggests an air embolism and should be so treated.

A diver who, while conscious, is passing nonfrothy blood from the nose and mouth may be suffering from middle-ear squeeze or a bloody nose. A bloody nose may be the result of a too-strong effort to clear the ears, or sinus squeeze. Ear bleeding is often the result of a broken eardrum.

Treatment: If the bleeding can't be stopped, medical aid should be sought. Similarly, if serious injury is suspected, medical aid is necessary. Keep the victim lying down, to avoid the possibility of fainting, and elevate the feet. If the bleeding is from the head, apply direct pressure with a sterile dressing. Do not attempt to clean a head wound as it may cause increased bleeding. Do not apply too much pressure on the bone beneath as it may be fractured. Raise the upper part of the body, head and shoulders if possible, and do not bend the neck as it may be fractured. Once the bleeding is controlled, apply a bandage to hold the dressing in place and continue the pressure.

Apply a clean compress (sterile gauze) to any wound.Lacking sterile cloth, use the best and cleanest at hand. In the absence of cloth, use fingers or hand. Apply a compress as soon as feasible. If direct-pressure application fails to stop the blood flow, try pressure above the wound.

The illustration on the following page shows the common pressure points for arterial bleeding. *Note:* This method cannot be used to control bleeding of the head, neck and torso.

Elevating the wounded member will have the effect of decreasing the blood flow. The pressure points as shown are pressed with the flat of the fingers, not the tips. See illustrations. ˙

Arterial Bleeding

Vessels carrying the blood from the heart may be ruptured. Such bleeding will be in spurts and the blood will be bright red.

Venous Bleeding

This is a rupture of the vessel carrying blood back to the heart. The flow is steady and the blood is dark red.

Underwater Bleeding

In this case the injury may not be felt immediately. Arterial blood will not spurt and there will be a cloudy diffusion in the water. The color will show green rather than red.

Minor cuts and abrasions may not require any treatment other than preventing flow of blood into the water where it may attract predatory fish. When the bleeding cannot be stopped, the diver or swimmer should leave the water.

Pressure Points

Place the victim on back. Then, using straight arm as illustrated, place the heel of the hand over the pressure point. Usually a little pressure will be enough. If the bleeding does not stop, place the other hand on top of the first.

Do not apply arterial pressure to the wounds of the head, neck or torso. Once the bleeding has stopped, apply a bandage to the dressing with sufficient pressure to keep the bleeding stopped and at the same time to allow the blood to circulate beyond the wound. A pulse should be felt beyond the wound. Sometimes pulse checking beyond the wound may be physically impossible.

Prevention of infection is important. Touching the wound with a dirty cloth or hands may cause infection. In an emergency, however, it is important to first stop the bleeding.

Tourniquet

The use of a tourniquet can be dangerous. A tourniquet should be applied with caution, followed as soon as possible by a doctor's attention. Use this method only when all others have failed and the victim's life is clearly in the balance.

A tourniquet is a broad band of cloth placed just above the wound to cause all blood flow to cease. Make sure you do not use a narrow band or wire. Do not allow the tourniquet to touch the edges of the wound. If the wound is in a joint, place the tourniquet just above the joint.

- Wrap the tourniquet cloth tightly around the limb twice and tie an overhand knot.
- Insert a strong, short stick or other article that will not

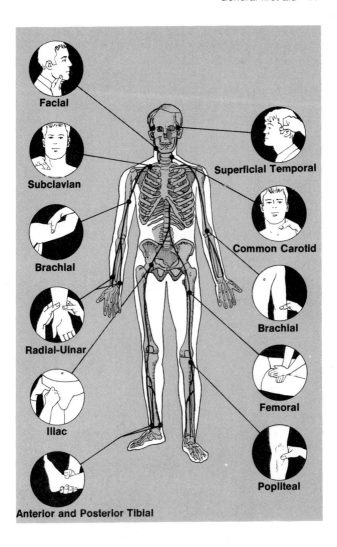

PRESSURE POINTS

break under the strain on the overhand knot. Then tie
two more overhand knots on top of the stick.
- Twist the stick and thus tighten the tourniquet until the
bleeding stops.
- Make sure the stick is secure and held in place with
the loose ends of the tourniquet.
- The limb with the tourniquet attached should be elevated.

See illustration on page 13.

SHOCK

Shock is defined as a bodily state resulting from de-
pressed functions. It may be more dangerous to the victim than the actual injury suffered. In some cases it may
lead to death.

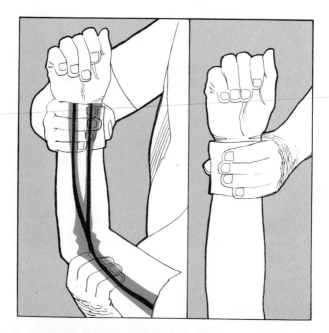

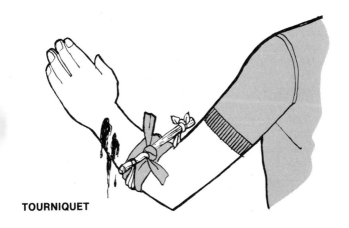

TOURNIQUET

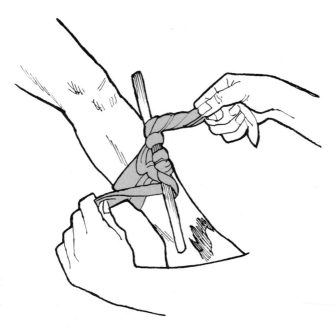

SECURING TOURNIQUET STICK

Symptoms: Rapid, weak, shallow breathing and cold, clammy sweat are symptoms of shock. The eyes are vacant and there may be nausea followed by vomiting. Pulse is rapid, weak and thready.

Treatment
1. Keep victim lying down; elevate feet.
2. Cover under as well as over the victim if climate dictates. This is to keep body heat from being lost.
3. Seek medical help immediately.
4. Take into account the kind of injury when making the victim comfortable.
5. If neck or spine injury is suspected, do not move the victim unless absolutely necessary. A rigid support un-

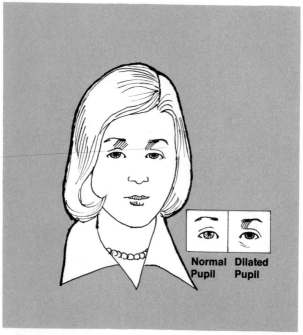

Normal Pupil   Dilated Pupil

LOOK OF SHOCK

der the back will prevent the injury from worsening.

6. When the injured person is suffering from serious injury to the lower portion of the face, place on side to prevent airway blockage and to permit drainage of collecting fluids.

7. When there are head injuries, be sure the upper torso (head and shoulders) is elevated. Do not elevate only the head as this could cause neck flexion and airway difficulties.

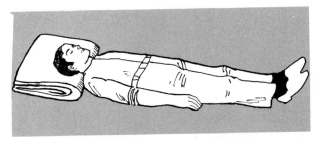

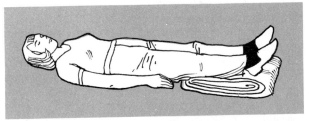

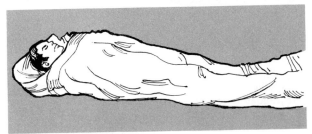

TREATMENT OF SHOCK

8. When there are no head injuries, the head may be kept lower than the feet.
9. Secure early medical help and call an ambulance if possible.

Providing Fluids to the Shock Victim

Do not administer fluids to an unconscious victim, when vomiting is present, or when abdominal injuries are suspected. When medical help is unavailable for over an hour and there does not appear to be sufficient reason for delaying the administration of fluids, tepid water may be given at the rate of about half a glass each 15 minutes. If nausea develops, stop giving fluids.

DROWNING

Cause: Asphyxia caused by lack of air.

Symptoms: Unconsciousness, not breathing, skin blue and discolored.

Treatment: Artificial respiration. Time is of the essence, as permanent brain damage may result if the brain does not receive oxygen for only a few minutes. Mouth-to-mouth resuscitation may be begun in the water. See below. If the heart is not beating, apply external cardiac compressions (CPR). Keep victim lying down and warm. Cardiac compressions can be given only if the victim is on a hard, firm surface. Secure medical help as soon as possible.

STOPPAGE OF BREATHING (ASPHYXIA)

Check for consciousness and breathing. Watch for a perceptible rise and fall of the chest. The pulse may be more readily noted by placing the tips of the fingers on the carotid artery located on the side of the neck.

The carotid artery runs along the side of the windpipe

and is easy to find using the tips of the fingers. It is more sensitive and easier to take a pulse from the carotid than from the wrist.

MOUTH-TO-MOUTH RESUSCITATION

Victim should be on back. Clear any foreign matter from the mouth. Use fingers wrapped in cloth if available. Watch that the tongue of the victim does not fall back and block the throat. To open the air passageway, place one hand beneath the victim's neck, then lift. Place the heel of the other hand on the forehead, tilting the head backward to its full extension. Try to keep the head in this posture as this clears the airway and moves the tongue away from the rear of the victim's throat. Using the thumb and forefinger of your hand on the victim's forehead, pinch the nose to prevent air leakage while you are expelling your breath into the victim's mouth; or you may press your cheek against the victim's nostrils. Open your mouth wide, take a full breath and seal your mouth, so there is no air leakage, around the victim's mouth. Blow into the victim's mouth four full, quick breaths initially. This may start breathing. About 12 breaths a minute for adults is right if continued resuscitation is required.

If the airway is clear, you should feel only minimum resistance. When you see the victim's chest rise, stop exhaling, remove your mouth, turn your head to one side and listen for the expelling of the air from the victim's lungs. Note the falling of the victim's chest.

When the exhalation is completed by the victim, repeat your cycle of blowing the air into the victim's mouth. If the victim has suffered damage to the mouth, you may blow through the nose. Close the victim's mouth, keeping the head in the same position. On the exhalation, you may open the victim's mouth to let the air out.

When using this method on children or infants, do not make the head tilt as far back as for adults. You may seal your mouth over both the nose and the mouth of the small

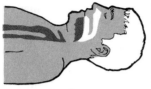

Airway Blocked

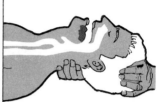

**Airway Straightened
For Mouth-To-Mouth
Resuscitation**

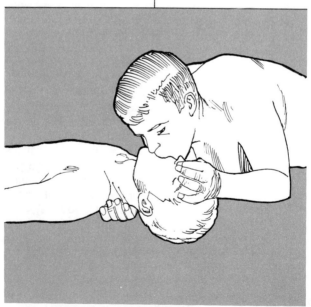

MOUTH-TO-MOUTH RESUSCITATION

child. Use about 20 breaths a minute, or one every three seconds, as opposed to 12 for adults. Small puffs will be adequate for infants. The objective is to have a rise and fall of the chest. If this does not occur there is something wrong. Check for blockage of the airway. Clear and continue with mouth-to-mouth assistance.

Continue mouth-to-mouth resuscitation until the victim can breathe without help. This may take considerable time. Cover the victim above and below to maintain body heat. Upon revival keep the victim quiet for about an hour. When victim can be moved, take to a hospital as a relapse might occur.

CHOKING AND STRANGULATION

Cause: Obstruction of airway by a foreign body, spasm, inhalation of vomitus or water; the crushing of the windpipe; the tongue falling back to block the airway.

Symptoms: Victim cannot speak, cough or breathe. The victim makes choking sounds; face turns blue; victim collapses into unconsciousness. Early recognition of airway obstruction is the key to successful treatment. *Note:* It is necessary to distinguish this emergency from stroke, heart attack or fainting, or other conditions that might cause respiratory failure or collapse. Foreign bodies may cause partial or full airway obstruction.

Partial Airway Obstruction

There may be good or poor air exchange.

When the air exchange is good, the victim can cough forcefully but there may be a wheezing sound between coughs. If the air exchange is good, the victim should be allowed to continue coughing and breathing effort. Do not interfere with the victim's efforts to expel the foreign body.

If there is poor air exchange, the victim makes a weak, noneffective cough and high-pitched noises while exhaling. There is increased breathing effort and possible cyanosis (blue hue to skin, fingernails and inside of mouth). At this point the partial obstruction should be dealt with as though it were a complete airway blockage.

Complete Airway Obstruction

The victim usually has been eating and suddenly is unable to speak, cough or breathe. The victim may clutch at throat. Quick action is required, preferably while the victim is conscious.

Back Blows: A series of rapid, sharp whacks with the hand over the spine between the shoulder blades. The blows should be rapid, forceful and delivered in quick succession. They may be delivered with the victim sitting, standing or in a lying position. While you deliver blows to the back your other hand may be on the chest to support the victim.

Victim Lying on Back (supine): Kneel and roll the victim onto side facing you with the chest against your knee. Deliver sharp blows as noted above.

Abdominal Thrust (Also Called the Heimlich Maneuver)

This is a series of rapid thrusts to the upper abdomen or chest in such a way as to force air from the lungs.

With Victim Standing or Sitting: Stand to the rear of the victim and wrap your arms around victim's waist. Put the thumb of your fist against the victim's abdomen slightly above the navel and below the rib cage. Grasp your fist with the other hand and pull toward you with a quick upward thrust. Repeat as required. This should expel the foreign body from the throat.

With Victim Supine: Victim is on back with the rescuer kneeling close to the side of victim's body, or astride victim. Place one hand on top of the other with the heel of the bottom hand just above the navel and in the middle of

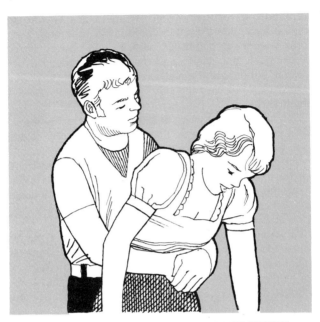

CLEARING FOREIGN BODY OBSTRUCTION OF AIRWAY

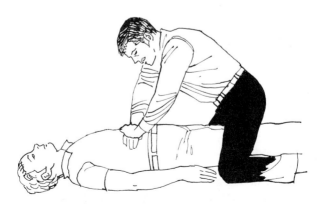

STRADDLE POSITION FOR CLEARING AIRWAY OBSTRUCTION

the abdomen, just below the rib cage. Rock forward so rescuer's shoulders are over the victim's abdomen. Then press toward the diaphragm with a rapid upward thrust expelling air and dislodging the foreign body. Do not press to either side. Repeat as needed.

Chest Thrust

This may be used when dealing with pregnancy, especially in advanced cases. Stand to rear of victim, place your arms under the victim's and around the victim's chest. Place the thumb side of your fist on the breastbone but not on the lower tip, or the edges of the rib cage. Grasp the fist with the other hand and exert a quick backward thrust.

Victim Lying Supine: Victim is placed on back. Rescuer kneels close to the side of victim's body. Place hands on victim's chest with the heels of the hands at the level of the nipples but not over the lower edge of the ribs. Apply a quick downward and inward thrust with a squeezing motion to compress the chest cavity.

HEART ATTACK

Symptoms: Pain in center of chest; substernal crushing sensation. Victim often experiences feelings of panic. Pain radiates to left arm, neck and sometimes the upper abdomen. There are symptoms of shock, such as excessive sweat and loss of consciousness.

First Aid: Allow victim to assume the most comfortable position for relief. It is usually not wise to force a patient to lie down. Loosen constrictive clothing, collar, belt. Do not lift the patient; do not supply anything to drink. Be steady and calm—call doctor and an ambulance. Be prepared to administer cardiopulmonary resuscitation (see page 23) in the event the patient loses consciousness, stops breathing and shows no pulse. Some patients with a history of heart attacks may have medication with them.

HEART FAILURE

Heart stoppage may be caused by a number of things, such as electrical shock, physical shock, respiratory accident or various medical conditions. Blood is not being pumped by the heart, and oxygen is not getting to the tissues. Brain damage can occur in only a few minutes.

Signs: Unconsciousness, lack of breathing, no pulse, no heartbeat.

Treatment: Cardiopulmonary resuscitation (CPR).

CARDIOPULMONARY RESUSCITATION

CPR is a combination of artificial respiration and artificial circulation. This should be begun immediately when cardiac arrest occurs. One should be trained in the process by either Red Cross or local Heart Society.

The brain is especially susceptible to damage when deprived of oxygenated blood. After six minutes' deprivation, the brain may suffer damage that cannot be reversed.

Three basic steps are involved:

A. Airway opened—by head-tilt method
B. Breathing restored—by mouth-to-mouth resuscitation
C. Circulation restored—by external cardiac compression

A and B constitute artificial respiration. C is artificial circulation. These three steps should always be done as soon as feasible. They should follow the sequence above.

Airway

Immediate opening of the airway is of paramount importance. Be sure the tongue is not fallen back and obstructing the airway. The head-tilt method will correct this. See illustration.

At times this is all that is needed to start the breathing cycle. The victim is on his back (supine). Rescuer puts one hand beneath victim's neck and the other on the forehead. Lift the neck with one hand and tilt the head backward by exerting pressure with the other hand. This extends the neck and lifts the tongue from rear of throat. Be sure to maintain the head in this position.

While victim is in this position, the rescuer should feel, listen and look to discover whether the victim is breathing. By placing the cheek close to the mouth and nose, one should be able to hear any respiratory sounds. While doing this, rescuer looks and feels for any rise and fall of the chest or abdomen. If there is none, the rescuer should begin artificial respiration. The description of artificial respiration is on page 23.

Artificial Circulation (External Cardiac Compression)

When sudden cardiac arrest occurs, the three basics of life support are needed in quick succession. The carotid pulse is felt for any sign of circulation. Absence of the pulse or very low pressure is a sign that cardiac compression is required to bring about artificial circulation.

External cardiac compression is the rhythmic pressure applied to the lower section of the sternum (breastbone). External cardiac compression should always be used in conjunction with artificial respiration. As noted above, artificial respiration is used first and then followed by cardiac compression. They should always be used together.

Technique for External Cardiac Compression

The victim is on a hard suface, face up (supine) and horizontal. Measure two fingerwidths from the lower tip of the breastbone (sternum). Care must be exercised not to put pressure on the lower part of the sternum.

Rescuer places the heel of one hand over the long axis of the lower portion of the sternum. The other hand is then placed on top of the first hand. The rescuer's shoulders are directly over the victim's sternum. The arms are straight. Rescuer rocks back and forth from the hips, exerting pressure downward and depressing the lower ster-

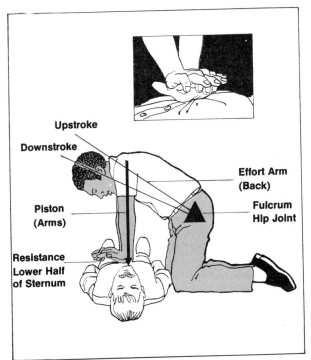

Upstroke

Downstroke

Effort Arm (Back)

Piston (Arms)

Fulcrum Hip Joint

Resistance Lower Half of Sternum

PROPER POSITION OF RESCUER AND VICTIM

num 1½ to 2 inches. The fingers of the two hands may be interlocked to help keep the fingers off the chest wall. Relaxation follows compression and is of the same duration. The heel of the rescuer's hand is not removed from the chest in the relaxation phase although pressure on the sternum is released fully. This permits the chest to return to its normal position before the next compression is begun.

Ideally CPR is best done by two persons, one doing the artificial respiration, the other performing external cardiac compression. The rate of compression is 60 to the minute when two persons are involved in the task. The rate of artificial respiration is 12 to the minute. One rescuer should be on each side of the victim.

Young children require ¾ to 1½ inches compression, while infants require ½ to ¾ inch compression. The rate for the young is 80 to 100 compressions per minute with breaths delivered after each five compressions.

Checking Effectiveness of CPR

Check the eyes during CPR and note if the pupil constricts when exposed to light. If it does, this indicates that a sufficient supply of oxygenated blood is getting to the brain.

WOUND CARE

There are two types of wounds—open wound and closed wound. An open wound is a break in the skin. A closed wound is an internal wound without an opening in the skin. Wounds are usually caused by an external physical force, such as falls, sharp objects, machinery or vehicular accidents.

The methods for stopping bleeding have already been discussed, but you should know about the care of wounds. Cleanliness is imperative. If possible, clean the hands thoroughly. Cleanse the wound. Boiled water and soap are good cleaning agents for this purpose.

Cover the opening with a dressing, preferably sterile. Be sure circulation can continue with the dressing in place. If a sterile dressing is not available, use the cleanest cloth you can find. Be watchful for redness and swelling and get the victim to a doctor as quickly as possible. Angry redness may mean bacterial infection. This can be caused by a nonsterile dressing or other dirt that has gotten into the wound.

Types of Open Wounds

Abrasions: Caused by scraping and damaging the skin. Blood ordinarily oozes from small capillaries and veins in such wounds. The danger here is of infection as dirt can get into the wound and cause contamination.

These wounds are often caused by falling or hard contact with rough objects. Examples are skinned hands and knees, rope burns and other injuries of this type.

Incisions: Commonly caused by sharp objects such as knives, scissors, glass, etc., which cut the flesh. Depth of such incisions will determine the extent of injury. Deep cuts may involve arteries, tendons, nerves and muscles.

Punctures: Caused by pointed objects such as knives, nails, pins, splinters, etc. Usually bleeding is limited to the surface. There may be more severe bleeding internally. Such wounds are easily infected, and tetanus organisms and bacteria grow in this type of wound where the blood does not flush. Antiseptics should be used with caution because of possible allergies.

Infected wounds demand prompt medical care. If there is an anticipated delay of any length before the victim will see a physician, here are some interim steps that should be taken:

1. Keep the victim lying down and immobilize the infected area to keep the infection from spreading.
2. Elevate the infected part of the body. This is important for infected wounds of legs, hands, feet and head.
3. Apply heat if possible to the area with hot-water bottles or use warm, moist cloths over the wound bandaging. Change these often to keep them warm. You may cover these with a dry towel wrapped in aluminum foil or waxed paper to hold the heat.
4. Continue with the warm packs for a period of 30 minutes; then take them off, covering the wound with a sterile dressing for 30 minutes. Repeat with warm packs again and follow with the sterile dressing again. Repeat this until medical help can be had.

This care should not impede the process of getting the victim to the doctor.

Tetanus: Its Prevention

Tetanus, or lockjaw as it is commonly known, results when the tetanus bacteria find their way into the body via an opening in the skin. Even small wounds can be dangerous because of the possibility of tetanus infection. Divers working in polluted water or mud may be exposed to tetanus. Particularly dangerous are puncture wounds as the bacteria are driven deeply into the body.

Protective methods consist of regular tetanus toxoid boosters every three years. Failure to maintain this schedule will mean that the attending physician will probably want to administer a tetanus booster shot. This may cause an uncomfortable reaction. You are well advised to keep your tetanus immunization current.

BROKEN BONES

The setting of broken bones must be left to the doctor. The important thing for the first-aid person is to know what to do. Careful handling is of primary importance. Wrong movements may seriously complicate the problem. Shock may not be avoided, but it can be reduced by proper treatment. Keep the patient warm and treat for shock. See page 12.

If bleeding is heavy, stop it by using the methods described under the section on Bleeding, page 8. Do not try to reset the bone or clean the wound. Rather, get the victim to a doctor quickly.

A splint is used to immobilize the break and reduce the possibility of additional damage. Any available material can be used as a splint—a diver's knife in scabbard, a folded magazine, a broom handle or a board, a folded wet suit, blanket or pillow. A splint should extend beyond the joint above and beneath a fracture. Move the injured member carefully when applying the splint. Place a hand on either side of the fracture in positioning it for splinting. Pad the splints if possible. Use whatever material is at hand for this.

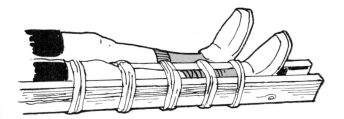

LEG SPLINT

Should the break be located in the head, neck, back or pelvis, do not move the patient without expert help. To do so may seriously aggravate the condition. Stabilize and immobilize the victim as found and prevent moving unless expert help is available.

Broken Neck or Back

Fractures of the neck may occur as the result of a fall or from a blow to the neck or head by a heavy moving object. The victim will complain of acute pain at the site of the fracture with a tingling or numbness. If the spinal cord has been damaged, there could be paralysis down from the site of the break. Severe shock accompanies the injury. This may be delayed for a time. Patients with neck paralysis may not be able to urinate. Medical advice by any means is necessary in the treatment of such patients.

A victim with a broken neck will not be able to move fingers or hands. If asked to grasp your hand, the grip will be weak. If the back is broken, there will be no movement of the feet or toes. If the victim is unconscious, it is possible to ascertain damage to the spinal cord by pricking the sole of the victim's foot using a pin or pointed knife. If the muscles of the leg are not paralyzed, the foot will be retracted quickly. If the leg muscles are paralyzed, the foot will be unable to move. Prick the victim's hands also. If the hand responds by jumping when pricked, the injury is below the neck (broken back). If there is no reflex jump of

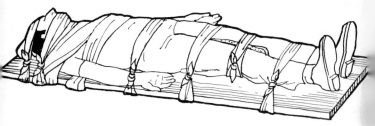

BACKBOARD FOR NECK, BACK, LEG AND PELVIS INJURY

the hand when pricked, the victim possibly has a broken neck.

Cover the victim to conserve body heat. Do not raise the head to give liquids. Get a doctor and/or ambulance with personnel who know how to handle a broken neck or back. Keep the victim from moving. Because of the possible involvement of the spinal cord such movement can result in paralysis.

If the victim has any breathing difficulty, the rescuer should follow the steps for clearing the airway. In doing this with a suspected neck injury, the head tilt should be minimal. Forward displacement of the jaw with positive pressure breathing should be done first if indicated.

If you must move a person with a possible fracture of the neck, the victim should be on his back for transportation. A body board to help immobilize the victim is important. It takes about three and ideally four persons to move such a casualty, and they should know precisely how to do it. They must know how to keep the victim's trunk and head as rigid as possible. No twisting, bending or side-to-side motion should be permitted while slipping a board or other rigid support under the victim. A towel may be slipped under the back of the neck and rolled-up clothing or blankets around the head, neck and shoulders to prevent movement. The victim is secured to the backboard by several bandages or ties.

If the helpers have not been trained, it is best to try the procedure on an uninjured person first. One person should steady the victim's head by spreading out the fingers and, with palms on either side of the victim's head and spread fingers reaching down toward the victim's shoulders, form a splint for the head and neck as they are positioned in the helper's hands.

In water accidents when the victim's neck seems to be injured, keep the victim floating by putting one hand under the shoulders and head. Try to keep the head from twisting or turning until a board or other rigid support can be secured. The victim must be lifted very carefully to boat or dock while in the support. An open airway along with respiration must be achieved during all of this.

Head Injury

Many diver accidents occur on the way to the water. Scaling a rocky embankment with a load of scuba gear may result in a fall.

Symptoms: Victim is dazed, possibly unconscious, bleeding from ears, nose or mouth, weak/rapid pulse, unequal dilation of pupils of the eyes. Sometimes paralysis is associated with the injury. This may involve legs and/or arms. There is double vision, temporary loss of consciousness and extreme pallor. (Or the symptoms may be very slight, only to appear later in a much more extreme fashion.)

Treatment: Dress wound(s). If patient is not conscious, allow the blood to drain from the mouth by turning the head sideways. Keep the patient lying down while you seek medical help. Get the victim to a hospital as quickly as possible.

Dislocated Joints

A dislocation occurs with severe wrenching or twisting of a joint. The ligaments holding the bones in position are stretched and may be torn, with the result that the bone ends are forced into an unusual relationship. Dislocations are usually caused by a blow or fall, or by very strenuous lifting, twisting or pulling where a sudden violent strain is placed on the joint.

Symptoms: Great pain, discoloration and rapid swelling accompanied by loss of use in the joint are apparent signs of dislocation. The joint is usually stiff and immobile and has an abnormal appearance.

Although a fracture and dislocation can occur at the same time, fractures usually occur between the joints. Joints most commonly dislocated are the shoulders and the fingers. The ankle joint is often dislocated and fractured simultaneously.

Don't move the joint. If the patient can be safely moved, get victim to a hospital as soon as possible. If the legs are involved and the patient cannot walk, make the victim comfortable and try to secure an ambulance. Cold compresses may help to relieve the pain and keep the swelling down.

Moving the Injured

Much harm may be done by inappropriate moving of a person suffering from a broken bone, particularly with a damaged neck or back. The well-meaning effort to get medical help at all costs may result in permanent injury or death to the victim. Do not move the victim until you have a clear idea of what the problem is.

When moving the injured person is vital to survival, move the victim in a reclining or semireclining posture. If you can make a stretcher from two poles and a blanket, do so; or use a strong board or other flat surface.

Avoid jackknifing the injured person into a car for transportation until you are certain the victim is not suffering a back injury or a broken rib.

BURNS

Classification: Burns are classified by depth, which may vary in severity in different areas of the body. Depth is noted as "degrees."

First-Degree Burns: These affect only the outer epidermal (outer skin) area and are characterized by redness, mild swelling, increased warmth, tenderness along with pain.

These burns are often caused by sunburn, scalding by hot water or steam; also sudden flash burns. Although quite painful, such burns usually heal within a week without scarring.

Second-Degree Burns: Such burns involve the entire layer of epidermis and extend into the under layer of the skin (dermis). Superficial second-degree burns are characterized by blister formation, deep reddening, much swelling and seeping of fluid. Second-degree burns are often indistinguishable from third-degree burns immediately following the injury. These burns are characterized by severe pain because of the sensitive nerve endings. Any pressure, breeze or disturbance to the area will cause increased pain. They can be caused by deep sunburn, scalding fluid and flash burns, as from kerosene or gasoline. If they do not become infected, they should heal with almost no scarring in about three weeks. If infection does result, the burn will transform into a third-degree-type burn.

Third-Degree Burns: These burns involve the epidermis, dermis and may also include the underlying fat, bone and muscle. They include charring of the skin. This may be black or dark brown, hard, cherry red and dry, milk white, thick and leathery. Coagulated blood vessels are frequently noted. Pain may be absent because of the destruction of nerve endings. Such burns are caused by hot liquids, ignited clothing, electricity, explosions and oil or gasoline fires. These burns will not heal properly by themselves, except at the edges of the wound. Skin grafting must be done early to avoid severe contractions as scar tissue covers the damaged area. Critical burns require prompt examination and hospitalization because of the life-threatening effect.

Treatment

First-degree burns that involve only a small section of the body usually need little treatment. For relief of pain, cold water can be applied to the burn surface or the burned area can be submerged in cold water. Dirty areas should be cleaned gently with soap and water and left exposed to air or covered with a clean, dry dressing. If sunburned areas are clean they should not be washed.

Second-Degree (small) Burns: For pain relief and the reduction of blister formation, cold-water applications should be used, or the burned area of the skin should be immersed promptly in cold water from one to two hours. Salt reduces the temperature of ice water and never should be added as it might cause additional injury. Following the cold treatment, the area should be cleansed gently with soap and water, then carefully blotted dry with sterile gauze or a clean towel.
- Do not break the blisters.
- Do not attempt to remove pieces of body tissue that adhere to the wound.
- Apply sulfadiazine silver cream 1% to the burned area and wrap with a sterile dressing. Remove the dressing daily and reapply the medication to the new dressing.

If the dressing develops an odor or becomes soaked with body fluids, it may be changed more often. When the dressing needs changing it should not be pulled from the adhering surfaces. The area should be soaked with large quantities of water to free the material from the wound. Before a new dressing is placed over the wound it should be washed gently with soap and water and sulfadiazine silver cream 1% should be applied.

First- and Second-Degree (more extensive) Burns: When first- and second-degree burns cover 15% or more of the body surface of an adult, the victim may require hospitalization. Burns that involve the hands, face, feet and groin area should be considered serious. Plans for the evacuation of such patients to a nearby medical facility are of great importance.

Second- and Third-Degree (major) Burns: (On more than 30% of the body surface of adults and children) Check the victim promptly for breathing and establish an open airway. Artificial ventilation and cardiopulmonary resuscitation should be given as needed. See page 23.

When there are burns about the face, head and neck, or if during the fire the victim was caught in an enclosed area, respiratory problems should be anticipated. Oxygen, if available, should be administered to major burn victims with breathing difficulties. Injury to the respiratory tract might have been done by the inhalation of smoke and other products of incomplete combustion. Carbon monoxide poisoning may also accompany the burn. These problems may not be immediately noticeable but will surface later when the membranes begin to swell because of inflammation.

While there may be no immediate signs of shock, it is due. Before local therapy to the burn is initiated, you should treat for shock. See page 12.

If the patient is not vomiting and is conscious he may take a weak solution of sodium bicarbonate and salt (½ teaspoon of baking soda and 1 teaspoon of salt to a quart of water). Take slowly by mouth. The solution should be at room temperature.

Dosages: An adult should be given approximately ½ glass each 15 minutes; a child, ¼ glass; and an infant, ⅛ glass. If vomiting occurs, discontinue the fluids immediately.

In treating a burn be sure to wash your hands thoroughly. If sterile gloves are available, put them on. All debris around the burn should be removed. Do not open blisters or try to remove pieces of burned tissue. Do not apply ice water to extensively burned surfaces. It may increase the victim's shock reaction.

After the burned area has been cleaned and the sulfa-diazine silver cream applied, many layers of sterile dressings should be added to absorb the copious fluids produced. If sterile dressings are not available, a freshly laundered sheet can be used. If adhesive tape is used to fasten the bandage, it should be kept off the skin.

Dressings should be left in place for 24 hours unless they become soaked with drainage. Fever following serious burns is common and does not necessarily indicate infection.

When treating for burns always check for other injuries. If there are fractures and lacerations, they should be treated the same way one would treat them if burns were not present.

Electrical Burns

The intensity of electrical burns is often difficult to determine because deeper layers of skin, muscles and internal organs might be involved. Such burns may be followed by a paralysis of the respiratory center with an irregular heartbeat. Unconsciousness or instant death may occur.

Treatment: The victim must be removed from the electrical current as speedily as possible without endangering the rescuer. Electrical lines may be removed with a wooden pole, chair or other nonmetallic object. Cardiopulmonary resuscitation (see page 23) may be necessary because of the shock to the victim's heart and lungs. The treatment of the burn is the same as for any burn of the same extent and depth: prevention and treatment of shock, care of the wound and control of infection.

Chemical Burns

Such burns occur when acids, alkalis and other corrosive chemicals come in contact with the skin and mucous membranes.

Treatment: The chemical must be washed away promptly with copious quantities of water. Use a shower or hose if available. The washing should continue for about five minutes minimum. The victim's clothing which has become contaminated with the chemicals should be removed. This washing technique should be modified for dry lime and carbolic acid burns. Water mixed with lime reacts to produce heat, which may further burn the skin. Before washing, brush the lime away gently. Carbolic acid crystals should be washed from the skin with ethyl alco-

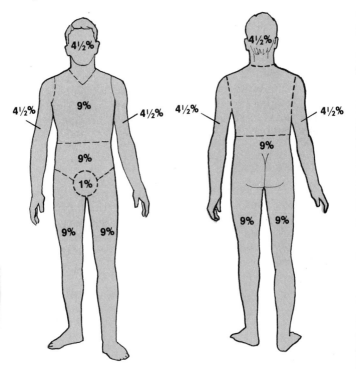

RULE OF NINES TO DETERMINE EXTENT OF BURNS

hol or isopropyl alcohol, then the skin washed with water. After thorough washing, any chemical remaining should be neutralized carefully. If the appropriate antidote is not known, perhaps medical advice may be had by radio. Additional treatment would be the same as for any thermal burn of the same depth and extent.

Extent of the Burn

The area of burned surface in an adult can be estimated by using the rule of nines. The head and neck represent 9% of the body surface, each arm 9%, the chest 9%, the upper back 9%, the abdomen 9%, the buttocks and lower back 9%, the front of each leg 9% and the crotch and genitalia 1%. In children the head is larger in relation to the body and should be counted as 18%. Except for this the basic rule may be used. An adult with 15% or more of second-degree burns should be hospitalized. Children with 10% or more of body surface burned require hospitalization because of the life-threatening nature of such an injury.

ELECTRIC SHOCK

Remove the victim from the electricial source as soon as possible. Rescuer should avoid contact with the electrical source to avoid becoming a victim also. Use a dry, nonmetallic pole, rope or even clothing to remove victim from wire or electrical contact. Rescuer should be on a dry surface, touching only dry materials that are themselves nonconductive.

Check for breathing and pulse and apply artificial respiration (mouth-to-mouth) and CPR if necessary. See page 17.

FAINTING

Arrange victim on back, keep the head low to bring blood to the head. Be sure the airway is clear. Loosen clothing, make comfortable. Upon revival, a cup of hot tea or coffee will help.

If unconsciousness persists, call an ambulance while keeping the patient warm, or if convenient, get the patient to a hospital emergency section.

Cause: Varied. It may be severe emotional upset, extreme fatigue, poor ventilation or shock.

Treatment: If the patient feels faint, sitting and putting the head between the knees usually will help. Or else have the patient lie down.

EXTERNAL EAR INFECTION

Cause: Bacteria most frequently cause swimmer and diver ear infections. Fungus in the ear is usually caused by high humidity, especially in the tropics.

Symptoms: Itching in ear, with pain; crusting in the ear canal; excretion of fluids from the ear canal; redness and swelling around ear.

Treatment: Keep ears clean and dry. Following a dive, irrigate ears for five minutes with Domeboro Solution, made by Dome Laboratories. Dry the outer canal following the use of Domeboro Solution. When an infection develops, see a doctor. Avoid poking in ears.

POISONING BY MOUTH

When anyone swallows poison it is a medical emergency. Every nonfood substance should be considered a potential poison. Take the following steps:

1. Try to determine the nature of the poison and the amount swallowed. Assess the patient's condition carefully.
2. If the poison container is available, read the label for

the poison ingredients. Often the poison antidote is also printed on the label.
3. If radio is available, use it for medical advice. If at sea this is the only possibility.
4. While waiting for medical advice keep the victim warm.

Swallowed Poisons

Make the victim vomit, but recall that there are conditions in which the victim should not be made to vomit. Do not make the victim vomit when:

- Victim is unconscious or convulsing.
- The poison swallowed is a strong corrosive, such as acid or lye.
- The swallowed poison contains kerosene, gasoline, lighter fluid, furniture polish or other petroleum distillates, unless so instructed by radio.

(Exception: If these are mixed with dangerous insecticides, then the poison must be removed.)

Directions for Making the Victim Vomit

Administer two tablespoons of syrup of ipecac to the victim. Follow this with one to two cups of water. If no vomiting occurs within 20 minutes, the dose may be repeated one time only. To induce vomiting, gently tickle the back of the throat with a spoon or similar blunt object.

Activated charcoal, two to four tablespoonfuls in a glass of water, may be given following vomiting, or if ipecac has failed to induce vomiting within an hour. Do not give activated charcoal before ipecac has had an opportunity to cause vomiting. Activated charcoal is safe to use and will bind a large number of poisons, preventing them from being absorbed into the body. Do not use the universal antidote: a mixture of tannic acid, charcoal and magnesium oxide. Formerly considered a general antidote, this should not be used because it is not effective.

Poison Contact of Eyes or Skin

Wash and flush thoroughly with water.

When Poison Is Inhaled

Remove the victim from exposure to fumes. Support respiration.

Important: Under no circumstances should liquids be given to a victim who is unconscious or convulsing.

Antidote: This is a substance which neutralizes the effects of a poison or prevents its absorption.

POISONING BY PLANTS

When exposed to the common varieties of poison plants such as ivy, oak or sumac, wash the contacted areas promptly with cold water and soap. Do not scrub; be gentle. Where itching has begun, pat on calamine lotion to reduce the aggravating itch. See a doctor if the condition persists.

APPENDICITIS

Appendicitis is the inflammation of the appendix. The appendix is a small pouch attached to the large intestine in the lower right part of the abdominal cavity. The usual signs and symptoms of appendicitis are cramps or pain in the abdomen, with loss of appetite, nausea and occasionally vomiting. The cramps subside, but the pain persists and becomes localized in the lower righthand side of the abdomen. Nausea and vomiting usually decrease when the pain localizes. There may be a rapid pulse, fever, constipation or, on occasion, diarrhea.

A laxative should *never* be given any patient suspected of having appendicitis.

- Keep the patient on absolute bed rest.
- Keep an ice bag over the appendix area.
- Do not give anything by mouth for at least 24 hours or until severe, acute symptoms have subsided. Then give small quantities of liquids such as water, Jell-O,

broth or fruit juice. As the patient convalesces, this liquid diet may be changed to a soft diet which is continued until all symptoms subside.

If the symptoms do not subside, the appendix may rupture and peritonitis may develop. With peritonitis, the victim may show symptoms and signs of shock. See Shock, page 12.

With peritonitis, the area of tenderness along with muscle tenseness spreads to almost the entire abdomen. The muscles may become very rigid.

The above treatment should be followed while waiting for a chance to take the victim to a hospital and a doctor's care.

SPRAINS AND STRAINS

Sprain is injury to a ligament, joint or muscle tendon in the area of a joint. Though a dislocation or fracture is not involved, there is injury to blood vessels and a stretching and tearing of the tissues. Sprains are usually caused by violent stretching or twisting. The wrist, ankle, back and knee joints are most often sprained. Sharp pain and marked swelling are characteristic of this type of injury. Any movement of the joint causes severe pain. The victim is often unable to use the joint. The skin may be discolored because of bleeding of torn tissues.

It is frequently difficult to distinguish between a sprain and a fracture. The injury should be treated as a fracture until the advice of a physician may be had or the victim's improvement reduces the possibility of a fracture.

Serious sprains often require complete bed rest from two days to a week. If the sprain includes the arm and shoulder, it should be put up in a sling. If the hip, leg or thigh is involved, the injured leg should be elevated by placing a pillow or a folded blanket under it. A patient with severe back sprain should be placed on his back with a board under the mattress, or victim should be on a straight, hard surface. A severe sprain of the lower back indicates that the victim should not stand or walk for several days after the injury, or until the pain has subsided.

Ice bags and cold wet compresses should be applied to the injured area for purposes of controlling swelling and for the relief of pain. For very severe pain, aspirin may be given.

The injured joint should be immobilized, utilizing whatever is available. On a boat—pillows, blankets, or with diver—wet suits, etc. An elastic bandage is helpful. The bandage should be applied firmly but not tightly. Check fingers and toes periodically for blue or white discoloration. This will indicate that the bandage is too tight. Pain, tingling, loss of sensation as well as loss of pulse means the bandage has been put on too tightly and needs to be loosened.

Strains

A strain is an injury to a muscle or tendon caused by sudden, forcible overstretching brought on by vigorous muscular effort. Running, jumping or heavy lifting can all cause strains. Back muscles are involved more often than leg or thigh muscles. Strains usually occur over the mid portion of the long bones rather than the joint.

Such injuries are characterized by pain, weakness, stiffening and knotting of the muscles (charley horse). Discoloration will often be noted because of blood seeping from the injured vessels into the tissues.

The injured member should be rested in a position comfortable to the patient. Moist heat, preferably, should be applied to the injury. This will relax the muscle spasms. Pain may be relieved and circulation stimulated by rubbing. It is frequently difficult to distinguish between a sprain and a strain. When in doubt, treat the injury as a sprain for 24 to 48 hours.

NOSEBLEED

Nosebleeds may occur as the result of an injury, a disease such as hypertension (high blood pressure), high-altitude exposure and overactivity or strenuous exercise.

Most nosebleeds are not serious and may be readily treated.

If the nose is broken, the victim should be taken to a medical facility as soon as feasible. Unless the broken nose is properly aligned the victim may have trouble breathing.

Treatment: The victim should be in a sitting position leaning forward. If the patient cannot lean forward and must be in a reclining position, the head and shoulders should be raised. Pressure is applied to the bleeding site and cold compresses applied to the nose and face. If the bleeding continues, a small gauze dressing should be placed in the nostrils and pressure applied. Leave a corner of the dressing protruding from each nostril for easy removal. A cold compress on the back of the neck will sometimes help. The victim should be quiet and not blow the nose for an hour or more after the bleeding has stopped. If the bleeding cannot be stopped, medical advice should be sought by radio or other means.

STINGS AND BITES

An insect bite or sting produces an open wound in the skin. The venom injected under the victim's skin will often cause local discomfort with swelling, itching or redness. Allergic reactions vary from a minor condition to anaphylactic shock. Those persons extremely sensitive to venom may not live an hour unless treatment is given promptly. Anyone who receives a bite or sting should be observed over a one- to two-hour period for any reaction.

Treatment: The stinger should be removed with tweezers if it is in place, as the venom will continue to be released slowly from the stinger if left in the skin. When minor allergic reactions are observed, the wound should be cleaned with soap and water. Cold applications should be used to reduce the swelling.

When required apply artificial respiration. Place the victim in such a position that the bite area is lower than the heart. Application of a restrictive band on the arm or leg above the bite and between it and the victim's heart will help slow the spread of the venom. Do not tighten the band excessively.

Get medical help as soon as possible if there is a severe reaction. If medical help is not available, do not leave the band in place over half an hour. If available, antihistamines may be taken in the prescribed dosage. Calamine lotion will help relieve itching.

Since some persons are violently affected by stings, they should be taken quickly to the nearest hospital for professional treatment. While on the way they may be helped by cold compresses and antihistamines.

Treatment for Minor Stings and Bites: Apply cold packs around sting site. Use calamine lotion for its soothing effect; other soothing lotions may also be used. For tick bites, covering the tick with heavy oil—even engine oil will do—should cause it to withdraw. Remove the tick with tweezers, making sure all parts are removed. Wash the area with soap and water. A gentle scrubbing action should remove all disease germs.

Aspirin may be used to relieve the pain. When multiple stings are involved, soak the victim in a cool bath, adding baking soda in the ratio of one tablespoon to each quart of water.

Scorpion

Scorpions have a stinger in the tail through which they inject venom.

Symptoms: Severe pain at the sting site; nausea and vomiting; abdominal pain, shock, convulsions and coma may result.

Treatment: Apply cold packs directly to the bite area.

Cold towels will do. A pad soaked in alcohol (30% by volume) combined with antihistamines is very helpful. Keep victim lying quietly.

Spiders

The black widow spider and the brown recluse are the most common poisonous spiders in the United States.

Black Widow Symptoms: Modest reaction locally; severe pain resulting from nerve toxin; heavy sweating and nausea; painful abdominal muscle cramps. A severe, cramping muscular pain spreads within an hour to the chest, abdomen, back and leg muscles. The victim may have a headache, difficulty in speaking and may be restless and perspiring.

Treatment: The wound should be washed with soap and water and a dressing applied. Apply cold packs to the bite area. Give aspirin for the relief of pain. If the allergic reaction is severe call a physician.

Brown Recluse Symptoms: Strong local reaction from the venom; nausea, chills, fever, vomiting and pains in the joints. If left untreated a rash may develop in a day or two; an open ulcer forms within one or two weeks. Blood changes may occur with the destruction of red cells. While these long-term changes should be noted and medical help should be sought, the immediate first aid should be as follows.

Treatment: Same as for bites of the black widow. Medication often fails to prevent extensive necrosis (death of tissue) and gangrene. It is necessary to get the victim to professional medical help to relieve the pain and other symptoms.

Tarantula: The tarantula spider inflicts a painful wound. See treatment for black widow and get the victim to a doctor as soon as possible, as the bite of a tarantula can

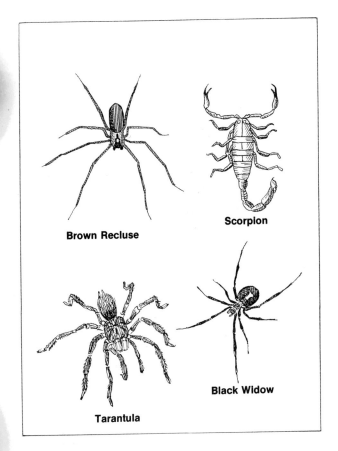

Brown Recluse

Scorpion

Tarantula

Black Widow

cause the death of tissue around the wound as well. Young children are in mortal danger from the tarantula.

The spider comes to the United States from South America and is often found in banana shipments.

SNAKEBITES

There are four major poisonous snakes in the United States. These are: rattlesnakes of many varieties, mocca-

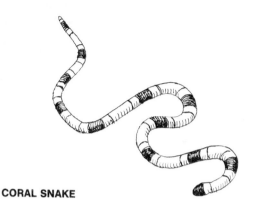

CORAL SNAKE

sins, copperheads and coral snakes. The first three are known as pit vipers. This is because of the small deep pit between the nostril and the eye on each side of the head. No nonpoisonous snake has this feature. The bite of the pit viper leaves a distinctive kind of bite pattern. This can be distinguished from the bite of a nonpoisonous snake. Thus, the victim need not be subjected to full treatment if the bite is nonpoisonous.

The bite of the pit viper leaves the clear marks of the fangs of the upper jaw—which make two puncture wounds at the point of damage. Additionally there are two rows of teeth marks from the upper jaw and two rows from the lower jaw. In contrast, the bite of a nonpoisonous snake leaves four rows of teeth marks from the upper jaw and two rows of teeth marks from the lower jaw.

The coral snake is quite small and marked with bands of red and black and narrow bands of yellow. When this snake bites it hangs on and sinks the fangs in with a chewing motion. The venom is most toxic, much like that of the cobra, and attacks the nervous system.

A pit viper bite is followed by severe pain accompanied by a swelling and deep purplish discoloration of the skin.

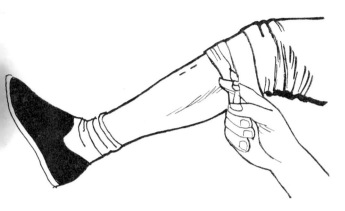

SNAKEBITE AND RESTRICTIVE BAND

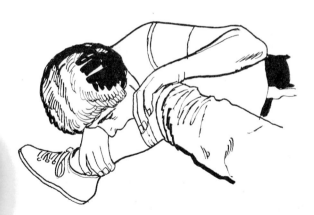

SUCKING VENOM

Usually the two fang marks are easily found, though if the victim was bitten on the toe, perhaps only one of the fangs had an opportunity to get in.

Treatment: The object of the first aid is to reduce the circulation of the poison in the area of the bite. The victim should not walk or move the affected parts. Medical assistance should be obtained as soon as possible. Constant reassurance is necessary for the victim.

Immobilize the limb in a lowered position and keep the area involved below the heart level. If the bite is on the arm or leg, tie a constricting band two to four inches above the bite, making sure the band is between the wound and the heart. This will decrease the flow of lymph from the involved area. The band should be snug but loose enough to allow a flow of blood into the limb. With a properly adjusted band there will be some oozing from the wound. Using a knife blade or razor, make an incision after the blade has been sterilized by flame. Make the incision through the skin only and in the long axis of the limb. Too-deep incisions may injure nerves or muscles. Be especially careful on the hands, wrists or feet as the nerves, tendons and muscles lie quite close to the surface. Make the incision no more than ½-inch long.

Apply suction with a snakebite kit if you have one, or suck the poison out by mouth, spitting out the contents of the mouth frequently. Continue sucking from 30 to 60 minutes.

- Wash the wound with soap and water and blot dry.
- Apply a clean bandage or sterile dressing and bandage in place.
- A cold compress may be used, or ice wrapped in a cloth may be placed over the wound to slow absorption. Do not pack the wound in ice.
- Do not give any alcohol to the victim as it will increase absorption.
- Treat for shock. Unless nausea and vomiting develop you may give the victim limited fluid if he can take it without difficulty.
- Watch for breathing difficulty, especially if a coral snake bite has been received. Apply artificial respiration if indicated.

- If the victim is alone and must walk, it should be done slowly.
- Even if the bite is from a nonpoisonous snake, see a doctor for antibiotic help and possible tetanus prevention.
- Get medical help as soon as possible. Call ahead if you can.

ANIMAL AND HUMAN BITES

Animal or human bites may cause puncture wounds and lacerations. There is immediate need to care for such wounds and prevent infection, especially rabies. Tetanus is an additional danger of bites. Rabies is carried in the saliva of the infected animal and treatment for this should be by a medical practitioner.

Treatment: Wash the wound thoroughly with soap and water. Be sure to flush it well. Apply a dressing. Movement of the arms and legs should be avoided prior to medical care.

CHILLING/HYPOTHERMIA

Hypothermia is a subnormal temperature within the body core. Research in the recent past has shown how dangerous this can be. Most boating deaths are now attributed to hypothermia. The drop in body temperature may cause the victim to lapse into unconsciousness or may even cause heart failure.

Symptoms: A hypothermic victim will have a blue-gray coloration with bluish lips. The body in an effort to conserve heat shuts down the blood vessels close to the surface. Breathing will be slow and labored, movements stiff and uncoordinated. The ability to use the hands and feet will be very reduced or lost entirely.

Cold-water immersion can cause hypothermia. The

skin and nearby tissues cool quickly. It may take 10 to 15 minutes before the brain and heart temperatures drop. A decline to 90° from the normal 98.6° can cause unconsciousness. A body temperature of 85° usually means heart failure or death.

A hypothermia victim should not be allowed to walk. Move the victim to shelter and warmth as soon as possible. Gently remove wet clothing. Place the victim on a hard, flat surface. Wrap warm, moist towels or other fabric around the head, neck, sides and groin. As the packs cool, warm them by adding warm water (about 105°). Heated blankets and hot-water bottles can also be used. In cases of mild hypothermia, shelter and dry clothing may be all that are required. Get the victim to a doctor as soon as possible.

A hypothermia victim should never be considered dead even if all signs of life are absent—no pulse, no blood pressure, pupils of the eyes fixed and dilated. Administer cardiopulmonary resuscitation. Hypothermia may increase the time until irreversible death of cells occurs. A hypothermia victim should be pronounced dead only by a doctor and only after the victim has been rewarmed and still does not respond. There have been cases of revival after 40 minutes. This has been especially true of children, although adults have also been revived.

Those hypothermia victims who have been cooled over many hours present special problems. Their rewarming is best left to a physician or a paramedic who can administer medication and start intravenous fluid. In any case, be sure the victim does not lose more body heat. Because of loss of strength and a generally weakened condition of the heart, it is very important that the victim be handled as little and as gently as feasible. Rough handling and jostling may cause cardiac arrest.

A method of rewarming a hypothermia victim is for one or more rescuers to use their naked bodies to warm the victim's naked body. The use of a sleeping bag or blanket to trap the body heat is important.

When the victim is breathing, using the warmth of the rescuer's exhaled breath can help. The rescuer has to breathe in unison with the victim. This coupled with the naked body method can help.

Wrapping the victim's head in a loose scarf or other covering will reduce the heat loss and additionally trap some of the heat in the victim's exhaled air.

Warm moist oxygen inhalation is a way of warming that has been quite successful. This is a special kind of treatment and may not be generally available.

Don'ts

- Do not give the victim any alcoholic beverage.
- Do not rub the body of hypothermia victims.
- Do not listen to a hypothermia victim telling you he is alright. Reason is the first casualty.
- Do not wrap a victim in a blanket without a source of heat with the victim. A blanket may insulate the victim's body from external heat and may distribute the core heat to the extremities, causing "after drop."
- Do not give liquid to a victim. He may draw it into the lungs, causing additional complications. Only in the case of mild hypothermia may liquid be given and then only hot, sugary liquids.

If a hypothermia victim is to be taken away by helicopter, be sure to shield the victim from the rotor blast as this will only increase the heat loss. Especially protect the head from heat loss.

FROSTBITE AND COLD EXPOSURE

Injury caused by exposure to very low temperatures varies and is determined by such factors as wind velocity, time duration of exposure, temperature and humidity. Wind and humidity in combination accelerate freezing. Cold dry air causes less injury than cold moist air. Wet clothing, alcoholic beverages, fatigue, emotional stress, smoking and wounds accelerate the harmful effects of the cold.

Symptoms: The signs of long exposure to extreme cold involve numbness, shivering, low body temperature, drowsiness, severe muscular weakness. In time mental confusion takes over. The victim staggers, eyesight is inhibited. The heart may go into fibrillation. Shock is evident. Death is usually attributable to heart failure.

Frostbite is present when crystals form in the fluids of the body, especially in the soft tissues of the skin. The problem increases if the injured area is thawed and subsequently refrozen. Frostbite is one of the more common injuries caused by exposure to cold. Usually the area involved is small and includes such areas as cheeks, nose, ears, fingers, toes.

Just prior to frostbite, the skin involved may appear slightly flushed. As the frostbite proceeds, the skin color will change to white or grayish yellow. Early pain is often felt but this subsides. Frequently there is no pain at all. The affected part may feel very cold or numb. Often the victim is unaware of the frostbite and only when a companion tells the victim is it known. It is difficult to readily ascertain the extent of the injury. Even after rewarming it is not possible to know the extent of the damage.

Damage to tissue usually follows the course of damage caused by burns. Superficial frostbite involves the surface area largely. It will look white or grayish, with the surface feeling hard while the area underneath will be soft.

With deeper frostbite, large blisters will appear on the surface as well as the deeper tissues. The area involved will be hard, cold and insensitive. When the various layers of skin are all involved, skin grafting may have to be done. When frostbite involves an area deeper than the skin, the destruction of the tissue can be severe. This is a medical emergency as gangrene may become a factor from loss of circulation to the injured part of the body.

Treatment: The first-aid objective is to prevent further injury, to warm the affected portion of the body and to maintain respiration. The best way to rewarm the injured part is with running or circulating water. If the part has been thawed and refrozen, it should be warmed at room temperature 70° to 74°. It is inadvisable to use excessive heat. This includes stoves, hot-water bottles, electric blankets and other electrical devices.

Frostbite
- Get the victim indoors as soon as you can.
- Give the victim a warm drink.
- Immerse the frozen part in water that is warm but not hot. Test the water by pouring some on the inner forearm. Mild temperatures are advised; slowly work up to 102° to 105°. If warm water is not available, wrap the part in warm blankets or a sheet.
- The frostbitten area should be handled gently. Do not massage it. As soon as the part becomes flushed, stop the warming process. Have the victim exercise the rewarmed part.
- Wash the affected area with water and soap or a mild detergent. Do not use laundry or dish detergent. Blot dry gently with sterile gauze or clean cloth.
- Do not break the blisters.
- If fingers or toes are involved put dry sterile gauze between them to keep them separated.
- Elevate the frostbitten areas and keep them from contacting clothing or the bed linen.
- If the victim must walk, do not thaw in advance. If travel is necessary, cover the affected parts with a clean cloth or sterile gauze.
- Give warm fluids if the victim is not vomiting and is conscious.
- Get medical assistance as soon as possible.

Prolonged Exposure
- Apply artificial respiration if required.
- Get victim into a warm environment as soon as possible. Remove cold, wet clothing.

- Wrap victim in blankets or place victim in tub of warm water.
- If victim is conscious, give warm liquids but nothing alcoholic.
- Dry the victim well if water was used to warm victim.
- Follow procedures listed under Frostbite.

EXHAUSTION SYNDROME

Cause: Excessive fatigue bordering on exhaustion may be the result of poor physical condition, cold water, or overexertion and panic.

Symptoms: Breathing shallow and rapid; air is moving in the upper portion of the respiratory tract with insufficient transfer of oxygen and carbon dioxide. A swimmer or diver may experience increasing difficulty just staying afloat. Swimming may become impossible, and the victim may collapse and become unconscious.

Treatment: Assist in relieving symptoms. Try to help the victim take long, deep breaths while you provide flotation or personally assist victim to stay afloat. Get to shore as soon as feasible.

HEATSTROKE

Cause: Overexposure to heat with a resultant rise in body temperature. Because damage to brain cells may result, prompt relief is important.

Symptoms: Body temperature rises, skin very dry and hot, rapid pulse, sudden collapse.

Treatment: Body temperature must be lowered as rapidly as possible. Sponge head and neck with cool water. Give the victim a weak solution of salt water at a ratio of one teaspoon of salt to a quart of water. Have victim see a doctor immediately following recovery.

MOTION SICKNESS

A major part of the inner ear is the three semicircular canals. They are a factor in equilibrium. They are filled with fluid. Any movement of the head causes a movement of the fluid in the semicircular canals. The movement of the fluid generates nerve impulses, which enable a person to make adjustments in position so as to maintain balance. The motion of a vehicle, whether ship, airplane, bus, etc., can produce nausea and dizziness. This is called motion sickness.

Fatigue, food or gastrointestinal problems may cause the person to be seasick. The victim may break out in a cold sweat and be subject to dizziness for a short period.

Treatment: The victim should be kept quiet and warm. Small quantities of dried food such as crackers, dry toast, bread or lean meat may be given. This may settle the victim's stomach.

The effects may be diminished by placing the victim in a reclining position with the head on a pillow and the eyes focused on a distant, fixed point.

Cracked ice may be given to help control vomiting and slake thirst. Do not give an excess quantity of liquids. There are motion-sickness pills which may be taken several hours before going aboard. These are usually cyclizine hydrochloride (50 mg taken by mouth). These motion-sickness pills may be given every four to five hours as required.

DERMATITIS

Contact dermatitis is caused by a reaction of the skin to external agents. These may be harsh chemicals or an allergy to food, drugs, etc. These reactions may occur on the first exposure or only after repeated exposures. The location of the involved skin is often a clue to the offending agent.

Itching is almost always present and skin eruption can

occur in either chronic or acute form. Acute contact dermatitis is often accompanied by redness, swelling, blisters. The blisters may vary from very tiny to inches across. Blister fluid is clear and the color of straw. The fluid crusts upon drying on the site of the original blisters. If the blister takes on the consistency and color of pus, this may represent a secondary infection of a bacterial type. Chronic low-grade contact dermatitis will often appear as only a slight redness with scaling accompanied by scratch marks or superficial cracks in the skin.

Constant exposure to salt water, particularly in the tropics and where there is no access to fresh-water showers, will cause dermatitis. When not treated it may cover the entire body, rendering the victim incapable of further swimming or diving.

Treatment: The victim should be removed from the area where the contact agent occurred. Remove the source of irritation by washing in fresh water to remove the salt. Dry thoroughly. Rinse diving gear in fresh water. Apply disinfectant powder to affected places. Avoid scratching the affected portions of the body. Do not wear clothing that aggravates the area involved.

During an acute stage, calamine lotion may be used to speed the drying of blisters.

EAR INJURIES

Ear Wax Impacted

The secretion of brownish wax in the canal of the external ear is normal. In excess, this can be a cause of deafness. Pain in the ear may occur when too much hard wax is accumulated.

Treatment: Hard ear wax may be softened by placing a few drops of olive oil or cooking oil into the ear and leaving it for 24 hours. Then it may be removed by gently

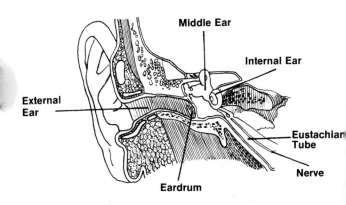

External Ear

Middle Ear

Internal Ear

Eustachian Tube

Nerve

Eardrum

syringing the ear with a solution of water and table salt (one tablespoon to a glass of lukewarm water). Ear wax should never be removed by forceful instrumentation. After irrigation, the external ear should be dried thoroughly with cotton-tipped applicators.

If the problem persists, the patient should see a doctor.

Another way to remove ear wax is to put a few drops of hydrogen peroxide in the ear and let it work for a few minutes. Then gently syringe the ear with plain warm water.

Earache

An earache may be caused by an infection of the middle ear; an inflammation, abscess or a boil of the external auditory canal; inflammation of the eustachian tube; dental conditions; mumps; and inflammation of the mastoid bone or nearby structures.

During a head cold or other disease, the ears frequently ache, feel sore or have a feeling of fullness. The same symptoms may occur when there is some other disease in which the respiratory passages are affected. Acute infection of the middle ear will cause severe earache and often results in the formation of an abscess.

Neuralgia is one of the causes of earache. It is characterized by a sudden stabbing pain. The victim feels as if someone had put a knife into the eardrum or the canal. Usually the pain stops suddenly. While the disease is fairly rare, it is important to know that not all sudden, stabbing, sharp ear pains are due to the most common causes mentioned earlier.

Treatment: The upper part of the ear should be pulled upward and backward to inspect the ear canal. Any redness, swelling or localized boil should be treated with hot, wet compresses applied over the ear. For pain, 600 mg of aspirin should be given by mouth each three to four hours as required.

Since symptoms similar to earache can be caused by dental conditions, the mouth and teeth should be inspected for dental defects. If the throat is sore and inflamed, it should be treated as described under Sore Throat, page 61.

Middle Ear Infection

Bacteria from the nose and throat reach the middle ear through the eustachian tube. Middle-ear infections ordinarily develop as a complication of a common cold, tonsilitis or an acute infection such as measles or scarlet fever.

Forcible blowing through the nose may drive infected mucus through the eustachian tube into the middle ear. A patient with nasal congestion should be instructed to blow the nose gently, preferably with both nostrils open. Acute infection of the middle ear often causes severe earache. It is usually accompanied by fever, and pus often forms behind the eardrum. If the eardrum is under great pressure, there is a throbbing pain. Spontaneous rupture of the eardrum with the release of pus provides dramatic relief from pain. If there are no complications, the infection clears up in about a week and the hole in the eardrum heals.

A chief danger from middle-ear infection is the spread

of the infection to the mastoid bone behind the ear. Mastoid infection is characterized by pain, tenderness or pressure behind the ear, continued earache even following rupture of the drum, and is accompanied by an increase in fever.

Treatment: For an infection of the middle ear an initial dose of penicillin V potassium, 500 mg, should be given by mouth followed by 250 mg every six hours. If the patient has an allergic reaction to penicillin, oral erythromycin should be used in the same dosage.

For pain, 600 mg of aspirin should be given by mouth every three to four hours as needed.

Chronic, low-grade inflammation of the middle ear without the formation of pus may be a complication of frequent and persistent colds. The usual symptoms are a nagging pain, a feeling of dullness or fullness, ringing in the ear and impaired hearing. This can be an important cause of loss of hearing and the patient should see a doctor.

SORE THROAT

A common complaint, sore throat may be just local or it may be part of a more serious illness. Laryngitis (inflammation of the voice box), tonsilitis (inflammation of the tonsils), and an abscess in the tissues of the tonsillar area are examples of localized throat conditions.

Streptococcal sore throat and diphtheritic sore throat are examples with marked systemic effects.

Pharyngitis and tonsilitis are common causes of sore throat. They frequently accompany a head cold. Pharyngitis may result from excessive use of the voice, too much tobacco or alcohol or mouth breathing. It may also be part of a more acute disease such as scarlet fever or "strep" throat. Such a septic throat may be very sore and accompanied by high fever and prostration.

Tonsilitis may lead to an abscess of the tonsil. This will

be indicated by a swelling on one side of the throat in the back. There will be great pain and difficulty in opening the mouth and swallowing. When the abscess breaks, these symptoms are relieved immediately.

A good light and a tongue depressor will allow one to see the condition of the throat.

Sore throat often begins with fever, malaise, headache, muscle pains and a slight chill. The throat feels sore, particularly on swallowing. Within a few hours the tonsils and throat are swollen, red, and the tongue coated. If the inflammation progresses, the patient may have difficulty swallowing.

Treatment: For simple tonsilitis or sore throat, gargling with warm saltwater (a teaspoon to a pint) every three hours may be all that is needed. Smoking should not be permitted. If fever is present, the patient should have bed rest. An ice bag applied to the neck may help. For pain, aspirin (600 mg) may be given every three hours. A liquid or soft diet is permitted.

SINUSITIS

During head colds or other respiratory infections, various microorganisms may transfer from the nose into one of the several sinuses through the small opening that connects these bone cavities with the nose. When the sinuses become infected and the mucous membrane is inflamed, the condition is called sinusitis. If the inflammation plugs the openings that drain the sinuses, secretions will accumulate in the sinuses, causing pressure and often fever.

This may be a temporary condition. As the infection clears and the sinuses drain, the swollen mucous membrane will shrink to its normal condition. Often the sinusitis becomes chronic. This means that there will be continuous local pain or discomfort, tenderness or pressure over the infected sinuses and a mild discharge from the nose.

Treatment: A patient with an acute attack of sinusitis should be put to bed. There will be pain and fever. He should be treated the same as for the common cold. To relieve the pain, hot moist compresses should be applied to the forehead, nose and cheeks. If sinusitis recurs frequently, the patient should consult a doctor.

COLDS

Symptoms of a cold are runny nose, watery eyes, malaise, aching muscles, chilliness, and frequently a sore and scratchy throat. A cold lowers a person's resistance to other diseases and allows for secondary infections. Cold symptoms may precede many communicable diseases. A cold may lead to bronchitis, pneumonia and middle-ear disease. Diphtheria, measles and septic sore throat may start as a cold.

Treatment: The patient should be kept in bed until the temperature is normal. Aspirin, 600 mg, should be given by mouth every three to four hours to help relieve the symptoms.

The victim should force fluids such as water and fruit juices. The victim should blow the nose gently to avoid forcing infectious material into the sinuses and middle ear. When the symptoms subside for a period of 24 hours, the patient may leave bed but restrict activity for a day or so.

RUPTURE (HERNIA)

A hernia is a protrusion of an organ or a part of the intestine through a wall of the cavity in which it is normally enclosed. Usually this means the protrusion of the intestine through a weak place in the abdominal wall.

Treatment: The victim should be placed on the back with the hips higher than the shoulders. The knees are drawn up to relax the abdominal muscles. By gentle manipulation with the fingers an effort should be made to gradually work the sac back into the abdomen. If the rupture has been protruding for a long time there may be adhesions which prevent its reduction.

When the rupture cannot be reduced, the protruding intestine may become compressed by swelling or adhesions to such a degree that the blood supply is cut off. This strangulated hernia is serious. Symptoms are akin to those of a bowel obstruction. Medical advice should be secured promptly, by radio if the boat is so equipped.

STROKE

A stroke occurs when the blood supply to some portion of the brain is interrupted. This is usually caused by:
- A blood clot forming in the blood vessel (cerebral thrombosis).
- A rupture of the blood vessel wall (cerebral hemorrhage).
- Obstruction of a cerebral blood vessel by a clot or other material from another part of the vascular system which flows to the brain (cerebral embolism).
- Pressure on a blood vessel, as by a tumor.

A stroke usually occurs very suddenly, without warning signs. In more severe cases, there is a rapid loss of consciousness with a flabby relaxed paralysis of the affected side of the body. Headache, nausea, vomiting and convulsions may be present. The face is usually flushed but may turn pale or ashen. The pupils of the eyes may be of unequal size. The pulse is full and rapid, while breathing is labored and irregular. The mouth may be drawn to one side and there is often difficulty in speaking and swallowing.

The symptoms will vary with the site of the lesion and the extent of brain damage. Mild cases may experience no loss of consciousness and paralysis may be limited to weakness on one side of the body.

Treatment: Following a stroke, good nursing care is essential. The victim should be placed in bed and undressed gently, with the trunk of the body, shoulders and head elevated slightly on pillows. Someone should be assigned to stay with the victim. Care should be taken that the patient does not choke on vomit or saliva. The head should be turned to one side to allow fluids to drain from the mouth. Food and mucus should be removed from the mouth with a cloth wrapped around a finger. If there is fever, cold compresses should be applied to the forehead. If the victim is conscious and able to swallow, soft food and liquids may be given. To prevent bedsores, the victim should be kept clean and turned to different positions in bed every three to four hours. Bowel regularity should be maintained.

Medical advice by radio should be sought as soon as possible, and early evacuation to a hospital is important.

TOOTHACHE WITH SWELLING

This is usually the result of infection by tooth decay. It may also be associated with disease of the gums. Frequently there is pain, swelling and the development of an abscess with swelling.

Treatment: For an infection, an initial dose of penicillin V 500 mg should be given by mouth, followed by 250 mg every six hours. If the patient is allergic to penicillin, oral erythromycin may be used with the same dosage and frequency. The patient should rinse the mouth with warm salt water, ¼ teaspoon salt to 8 ounces of water. This should be done for five minutes of each hour. This may produce early drainage and relief from pain. It also will cleanse the mouth and localize the infection. The patient should see a dentist as soon as possible. Aspirin may also relieve the pain. Oil of cloves on the tooth may relieve pain.

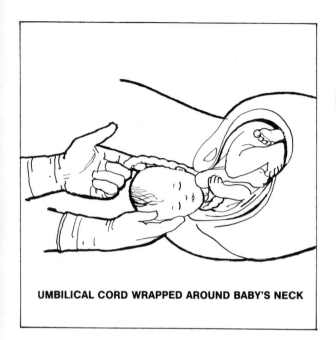

UMBILICAL CORD WRAPPED AROUND BABY'S NECK

EMERGENCY CHILDBIRTH

Just before birth there will be a discharge of amniotic fluid or the breaking of the bag of waters. This discharge is about a quart. The baby may follow quite rapidly. Have someone stay with the expectant mother.

Treatment:
- Call ambulance if possible.
- Have mother lie down.
- Keep everything as clean as you can. Wash hands, put a clean towel beneath the mother's hips for the baby to emerge on.
- If time permits, boil scissors and string for cutting and tying the umbilical cord.

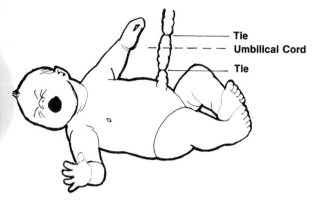

Tie
Umbilical Cord
Tie

TYING AND CUTTING THE UMBILICAL CORD

- Hold the baby gently as it emerges. Do not pull at all.
- If baby does not cry after being born, hold it upside down gently by its feet and slap it a couple of times on the seat.
- Wipe the baby's mouth clean of mucus by wrapping a clean handkerchief over a finger. If baby still is not breathing, use gentle mouth-to-mouth breathing.
- After the baby cries, place it on one side of the mother's abdomen with the face down and the head slightly lowered. Keep the baby warm by covering.
- When the baby is breathing regularly, look for the afterbirth to come from the mother. Do not pull on the cord.
- If there is time to sterilize the scissors and cord, wait for the doctor as there is no hurry. If there is no help on the way you may tie a strip from a clean handkerchief or even a shoelace. Wait until the cord stops pulsing before you tie it off. See illustration, above. Tie a square knot above and below the place where the cord will be cut.
- Do not handle the baby more than is necessary. If

there is bleeding, press a gauze pad against the area
to stop the bleeding.
Do Not:

- Hurry the birth.
- Interfere with the birth.
- Hurry to cut the cord. You can wait until the afterbirth is all out.
- Wash the white material off the baby as it protects the skin.
- Tamper with the baby's eyes, ears or nose.

Symptoms That May Spell Trouble

Get in touch with a doctor if any of these symptoms
occur. Let him decide what to do.

- Vaginal bleeding even if slight. The mother should go to bed and take nothing by mouth but water.
- Sharp and continuous pain in the abdomen.
- Chills and fever.
- Persistent headache, severe.
- Blurring of vision.
- Sudden discharge of fluid from the vagina.

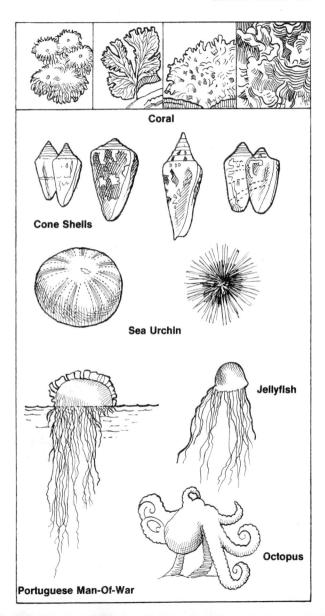

Coral

Cone Shells

Sea Urchin

Jellyfish

Octopus

Portuguese Man-Of-War

2
Injuries caused by marine life

Cause	Prevention	Symptoms	First Aid
Marine Plants	Avoid rapid entangling movements.		Go straight to surface, look for a clear area. Go straight down to clear area. Repeat till free.
Coral	Wear protective clothing: shoes, gloves. Avoid contact. Be aware of tidal surge toward coral heads.	Cuts, abrasions, welts, pain, and itching. Severe reactions are unusual.	Rinse area with baking soda solution, weak ammonia or plain water. Apply antihistamine or cortisone ointment. Antihistamine may be given by mouth to alleviate first pain and reaction. When pain subsides, wash with soap and water.

		cover with a sterile dressing. Refer stubborn cases to physician.
Sea Urchin	Avoid contact. The needlelike spines will penetrate dive clothing.	Prompt, intense burning sensation, followed by redness, swelling and aching. Irregular pulse may occur. In some instances, paralysis, respiratory distress and death ensue.	Remove all spines possible with tweezers or pliers. Clean the area. Cushion with loose dressing. Refer problems to a doctor, particularly removal of deeply imbedded spines.
Cone Shells	Avoid contact with soft parts of the organism.	Puncture wound. Loss of blood. Stinging, burning sensation. Numbness begins at wound and spreads quickly. In severe cases: paralysis, difficult breathing, coma, heart failure.	No specific care. Remove victim from the water. Keep victim lying down. Secure medical attention as soon as possible. May use hot applications.

Cause	Prevention	Symptoms	First Aid
Jelly Fish, Sea Nettles, Portuguese Man-of-War, Sea Wasp	Watch out, avoid contact. Wear protective clothing. Avoid touching dead ones.	Vary with species. From mild stinging to intense burning, throbbing, shooting pain. Loss of consciousness may occur. Skin will show welts, blisters, swelling, bleeding, shock, cramps, vomiting, respiratory problems, convulsions, death. The Sea Wasp may cause death in a few minutes.	Get buddy help. Leave water. Remove tentacles with cloth or seaweed. Use cortisone or antihistamine ointment to relieve pain. Secure medical help in severe cases. Where the Sea Wasp or Portuguese Man-of-War is involved, medical help is vital.
Octopus	Avoid tentacles. Cup action may be defeated by porous cloth. Avoid the beak at base of tentacles.	Bites induce swelling, heat, redness. Bleeding may be copicus.	Cold compresses to wound. Victim lying down. Secure medical help if bite involved. Use bleeding control technique.

| Sting Rays | Avoid treading on them in shallow water. Shuffle rather than step to avoid. Watch out for tail base barb. | Pain, fainting, weakness in less than 10 minutes. Pain may involve all of limb within $\frac{1}{2}$ hour. Maximum pain level in $1\frac{1}{2}$ hours. Wound may be puncture or laceration. | Leave water promptly. Wash with clean salt solution. Use clean, cold water. Remove any of the barbs still in wound. Soak in hot water for $\frac{1}{2}$ hour. Hot compresses are alright if a soaking is impossible. Get medical help if treatment fails to bring relief. Chest and abdomen wounds require medical attention. |

Cause	Prevention	Symptoms	First Aid
Venomous Fish: Horned Sharks, Catfish, Weeverfish, Scorpion Fish, Rabbit Fish, Rat Fish, Toad Fish, Zebra Fish, Sturgeon or Stonefish	If diving in a strange area, talk with local divers. Find out about harmful marine life.	Various symptoms. Usually puncture wounds. May be laceration type. Poison injected by spines causes swelling, redness, pain, muscle spasm, respiratory problems accompanied by convulsions. Death in severe instances.	Reduce pain, prevent a secondary infection, combat poison. Leave water promptly. Wash with clean, cold water. Make small cut across wound and apply suction. Soak in very hot water (avoid scalding) ½ to 1 hour. Epsom salts added may help. Cleanse further following soaking. Secure medical help as soon as possible.
Bite Wounds: Shark, Barracuda, Moray Eel, Orca, etc.	Avoid areas where predatory fish are found. Avoid splashing. Don't wear shiny articles, rings,	Bites cause lacerations with severe loss of blood. The wound is often jagged, of puncture	Control heavy bleeding promptly. See page 8. Get out of water. Treat for shock. See page 12.

		type. Often there is a tissue loss and deep shock.	Get medical help fast. Use constricting band. Watch respiration and pulse. Use AR/CPR if necessary.
Sea Snakes	Leave them alone.	Toxic signs appear in 15 to 20 minutes. Puncture type of wound. Malaise, respiratory spasm, respiratory distress, convulsions, shock, unconsciousness. Death in 25% of cases.	Leave water promptly. Place constricting band above bite to slow the venom. Do not loosen band. Keep victim at rest. Secure medical help promptly. The constricting band is not a tourniquet. Try to identify the snake. Cutting may be in order. See Snake Bites, page 47. Suction but not by mouth.

Cause	Prevention	Symptoms	First Aid
Eating inedible marine animals, poisonous. Too many to catalogue.	Check local divers and other sources before eating fish caught in unfamiliar areas.	Tingling about the lips and tongue. Vomiting, diarrhea, thirst. Poor coordination, numbness, paralysis, convulsions. Time frame up to 30 hours following eating of the fish.	Induce vomiting. Several glasses of warm, salty water will help. Add more water to cleanse digestive tract. Rash and welts may be relieved by a cool shower. If polluted clams or mussels are the cause of poisoning, baking soda added to the water is helpful. See a physician. If possible save samples of the vomitus and the food eaten for analysis.

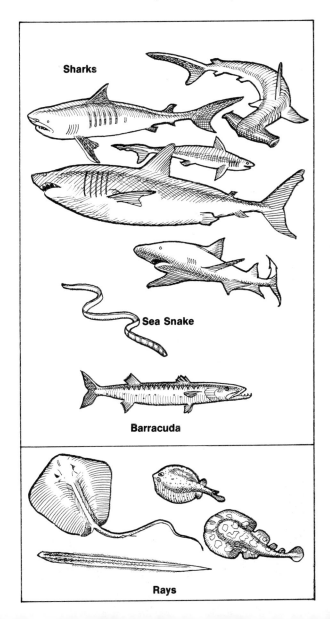

Sharks

Sea Snake

Barracuda

Rays

3
Pressure-related illness and injury

DECOMPRESSION SICKNESS

Cause: Also referred to as "bends" or "caisson disease," compressed-air illness is caused by insufficient decompression following a dive. With exposure to increased pressures, nitrogen has been absorbed into solution in the body tissues. If the diver surfaces quickly, reducing the pressure, the inert gas is released into the tissues and bloodstream in the form of bubbles. A controlled ascent allows the body to void the excess gas so as not to form bubbles but to remain in solution.

Symptoms: These vary and often are similar to those of air embolism. Symptoms occurring more than 15 minutes after surfacing, however, may generally be considered not to be from air embolism. Local pain and clumsiness, staggering, poor response, paralysis or partial paralysis, shortness of breath, blotchy skin, collapse with unconsciousness. Disturbance of vision and severe abdominal pain may precede abdominal hit.

Treatment: Recompression as soon as possible. Administer oxygen on the way to the chamber. This can be pure 100% oxygen. Most cases of decompression sickness will occur within three hours after diving. Of these, one-half of the victims will be stricken in the first half-hour. A very few cases, approximately 1%, will occur after six hours. Because pressure chambers are relatively few and far between, it is wise for the diver to note in advance the nearest available chamber. See introductory notes. Check for circulation.

AIR EMBOLISM

Cause: This is a result of the expansion of gas in the lungs usually caused by breath-holding on ascent. It can

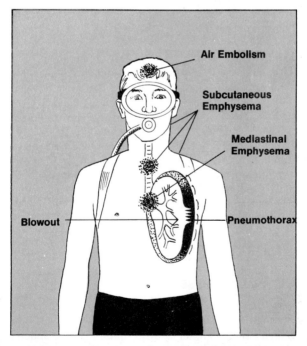

POSSIBLE CONSEQUENCES OF OVERINFLATION OF THE LUNGS

also be caused by failure to equalize pressure in the lungs. The gas expands as the surrounding pressure decreases; and, unless the gas can be breathed away, the lung tissue may rupture allowing bubbles to escape into the bloodstream. The bubbles tend to travel upward, and so they move toward the brain. As the bubbles reach smaller and smaller vessels, they finally stop, cutting off circulation. Serious damage can result in a very short time where the brain is involved.

Symptoms: These can occur within three to five minutes of surfacing. Dizziness, weakness, paralysis, blurred vision, shortness of breath, cough, sensation of a blow on the chest with progressive worsening, unconsciousness either before surfacing or immediately after, convulsions and failure to breathe.

Treatment: Prompt first aid. Place the victim on left side with head and chest on a downward incline. This will reduce the chance of bubbles reaching the brain. Breathing of 100% pure oxygen will also be helpful. If the oxygen is available, it may be administered on the way to the recompression chamber. Prompt recompression will reduce the size of the bubbles and permit blood circulation to resume. Do not attempt to take the victim back underwater to attempt treatment. When breathing has stopped, artificial respiration should be given promptly. If a tilt board is available, the feet can be elevated about 30°. CPR and oxygen should be given if necessary. The illustration shows what happens when air is released into body cavities as a result of excessive pressure.

MEDIASTINAL EMPHYSEMA

Cause: Can result from an injury to the lung, esophagus, trachea or bronchus. May not be serious but can signal an air embolism. Air is forced into the tissue spaces in the middle of the chest.

Symptoms: Include chest pain, trouble in breathing, trouble swallowing and shock.

Treatment: Recompression if it is serious; otherwise, rest and general medical care. Oxygen may be helpful.

SUBCUTANEOUS EMPHYSEMA

Cause: Air escapes into the tissues under the skin, usually in the area of the neck or collarbone.

Symptoms: Sensation of fullness in the neck region, change in the sound of one's voice, a swelling in the neck area, difficulty in breathing and swallowing, crackling feeling when skin is moved.

Treatment: Unless air embolism is present, recompression is not necessary. However, when in doubt always recompress. Give oxygen if available and see a physician.

PNEUMOTHORAX

Cause: Air has escaped from the lungs and lodged between the lung and the inner chest wall cavity. With the expansion of the air there may be either partial or complete collapse of the lung. When the case is serious, the heart may be displaced.

Symptoms: Shortness of breath; sudden development of cough, pain in chest aggravated by breathing; blueness in skin, fingernails, lips; rapid shallow breathing; a tendency to bend toward the side involved.

Treatment: Recompression will give temporary relief, but often the pneumothorax will need to be relieved by the insertion of a needle in the chest before the man can be brought up. This should be done only by a doctor. Prevention is the key word in lung accidents. As a cause of death in scuba diving, these accidents run a close second to drowning. Many cases are quite probably not recognized.

UNCONSCIOUS DIVER

A diver taken from the water in an unconscious state, or who becomes so upon leaving the water, should be treated as an air embolism case unless the cause is definitely known as something else. If breathing has stopped, use artificial respiration. Continue until breathing is resumed. Recompress the victim as soon as possible. Check for circulation.

SQUEEZE

Cause: Failure to equalize pressure differential during a dive. This can happen on either descent or ascent, but usually happens on descent. Most generally affected are the ears. However, squeeze can also happen in the sinuses, lung, face mask, teeth or gut.

Symptoms: The ears are most commonly affected, often the result of diving with a cold. The eustachian tube is blocked and equalization of pressure is impaired. There is pain in the ear; the drum may rupture, with bleeding into the external ear.

Treatment: Avoid diving until ear has healed. See a physician before resuming diving.

Sinus Squeeze

Symptoms: Severe pain in the sinus region around the eyes, bloody discharge from the mouth or nose, blood in face mask.

Treatment: None needed in minor instances. Stop diving and see a doctor.

Lung Squeeze

This is more of a hazard to the skin diver who holds his breath.

Symptoms: Sensation of compression in the chest during descent, chest pain. The diver may experience difficulty in breathing at the surface.

Treatment: If the case is severe, the diver may need help to reach the surface. Place victim face down and clear the mouth. Administer artificial respiration as required. If oxygen is available, administer it. Watch out for shock and treat if it occurs. Get medical attention quickly.

Mask Squeeze

Cause: Usually caused by failure to admit air into the face mask to equalize pressure on descent. The consequent pressure difference between the air pocket in the inflexible mask and the soft tissues of the face may result in tissue damage. The eyeballs and surrounding areas may also show damage.

Symptoms: The mask is pressed hard against the face; there is a feeling of suction and a painful squeezing. The face becomes bruised; the whites of the eyes turn red; eyeballs may protrude, with resultant bleeding behind as well as within the eyeball.

Treatment: Place ice packs on the damaged tissues, give pain relievers as necessary, and see a doctor as soon as possible.

OXYGEN SHORTAGE (HYPOXIA)

A serious and not uncommon hazard in breath-hold diving is hypoxia. This is a result of dangerously low oxygen levels and can cause loss of consciousness and drowning. In a normal dive, carbon-dioxide levels build up and force you to return to the surface, where you may resume breathing. This generally happens before the body's oxygen levels are dangerously lowered.

Unusually vigorous hyperventilation before a dive may mean trouble. Hyperventilation lowers the body's carbon-dioxide levels but does not add to the oxygen in any significant way. During the dive you may deplete your oxygen levels before you feel the urge to return to the surface. There is no warning signal, and a loss of consciousness can happen. No method of trying to extend the length of breath-hold dives is without risk.

Cause: Inadequate air supply. More common in closed-circuit scuba and semiclosed mixed-gas-type scuba. Body cells do not get enough oxygen to perform their normal functions.

Symptoms: Confusion, difficulty in standing or walking, poor coordination, blueness of lips and skin, drowsiness and sudden unconsciousness.

Treatment: Fresh air, oxygen, artificial respiration until consciousness is regained.

OXYGEN TOXICITY

Cause: Breathing pure oxygen under pressure. This is usually associated with closed-circuit scuba when the diver has exceeded safe depth limits.

Symptoms: Nausea, twitching of face, dizziness, hearing and vision problems, confusion, anxiety, unusual fatigue, clumsiness, convulsions.

Treatment: Bring diver to surface and remove source of oxygen. If the diver is convulsing, treatment follows this stage. If breathing has stopped, administer mouth-to-mouth resuscitation. When the diver is brought up during a convulsion and air embolism is suspected, get victim to a chamber as soon as possible.

CARBON-DIOXIDE EXCESS (HYPERCAPNIA)

Cause: The normal carbon-dioxide levels in the body are changed. Inadequate ventilation, with consequent buildup of carbon dioxide.

Symptoms: Severe drowsiness, confusion, muscle spasms, rigidity, unconsciousness.

Treatment: Fresh air, artificial respiration as required. Aftereffects are headache, dizziness, nausea with sore chest muscles.

NITROGEN NARCOSIS

Cause: The high partial pressure of nitrogen which becomes increasingly dangerous at depths over 100 feet.

Symptoms: Irresponsible, irrational behavior.

Treatment: Returning to shallower depths usually provides prompt relief.

CARBON-MONOXIDE POISONING

Cause: Carbon monoxide (CO) combines with hemoglobin and keeps the blood from carrying oxygen to the brain or other tissues. It may get into diving air sometimes from the engine exhaust, which is picked up by the air-compressor intake; or it may come from the lubricating oil vapor in the compressor.

Symptoms: At times a headache, dizziness and nausea serve as a warning before the carbon-monoxide victim becomes helpless. There is an unnatural redness of the lips and skin. *Note:* This does not occur in all cases. Other symptoms are similar to hypoxia: confusion, poor coordination, drowsiness and sudden unconsciousness.

Treatment: An unconscious carbon-monoxide victim requires pure oxygen and may be helped by increased oxygen pressure treatment. Access to fresh air is sufficient if the victim is breathing. If victim is not breathing, the treatment is the same as for drowning. See below.

DROWNING

Drowning is the most common cause of death in scuba diving. It is usually the culmination of a series of errors. Drowning is an asphyxia connected to the aspiration of fluids or the obstruction of the airway, which is caused by a spasm of the larynx while the victim is in the water. It is a major cause of death in the United States.

A scuba or breath-hold diver is prone to more risk than a surface swimmer or a hard-hat diver. So long as the equipment works, the diver is usually alright. It takes very little to set off a chain of events that can be fatal.

Panic is more often the prelude to scuba deaths than anything else.

Causes: Heart attack, stroke, overexertion. Fainting and even epileptic attacks can occur in the water as on land. Sometimes a head injury brought about by diving on a hard object can cause unconsciousness and drowning. Cramps in the various parts of the body can incapacitate a swimmer or diver so that he panics or cannot breathe. A reflex spasm of the larynx can result in a closed airway. Sometimes very cold water can cause this spasm. The victim may be subject to pain and fear as well. Loss of consciousness will often result, and the victim slips beneath the surface of the water. Because the airway is closed, the lungs may contain very little, or no water at all.

Hyperventilation can cause drowning of the skin diver when the carbon-dioxide level in the blood is lowered and no increase in oxygen is forthcoming. The victim may lapse into unconsciousness without warning and drown, as the mouth is opened and an inhalation aspirates water into the lungs.

First Aid: In the case of a scuba diver you may try mouth-to-snorkel breathing while in the water. Mouth-to-mouth resuscitation is difficult while you are trying to rescue the victim. The mouth-to-snorkel method allows the victim's head to be beneath the water while he is towed to shore and the air is getting into the lungs. This method should be learned because it is quite effective.

At any rate, artificial respiration should be started as soon as feasible. Treat for shock and get the victim to where medical care can be given. After the inflation of the victim's lungs with 10 quick breaths, move the victim ashore or onto a suitable flotation device, unless there is some evidence of injury to the neck or spinal cord which requires either a backboard or some other rigid support.

Keep the victim from becoming chilled. Continue artificial respiration.

Do not permit a person who survives a near drowning to walk. Delayed complications are most common. A victim should be observed for several days following the near drowning and this can be done best in a hospital. Cardiopulmonary resuscitation is an important adjunct to reviving an unconscious diver or swimmer. See page 23.

DIVING ABOVE SEA LEVEL

The U.S. Navy decompression tables are designed for diving in the ocean. Diving above sea level puts the diver at a lower ambient pressure and at greater risk of bubble formation. The tables were not composed for diving above sea level. If the tables are applied as given, diving in a mountain lake involves considerable risk. Some work has been done with modified tables, but thus far there has been no experimental validation for these. There is evidence that such small elevations as 600 to 800 feet may cause problems with some of the tables.

FLYING AFTER DIVING

Following a no-decompression dive, a diver will have significantly more nitrogen in the tissues than prior to the dive. Prolonged exposure to altitude may bring symptoms of bubble formation. A good rule of thumb is to wait 24 hours to fly following a dive.

ALCOHOL AND MARIJUANA

These substances are known to interfere with the capacity of the skin blood vessels to constrict and consequently may lead to a too-rapid heat loss from the body. This can bring on hypothermia. It is best not to indulge in either of these while diving.

4
The uses of boating and diving gear for first aid

EMERGENCY USE OF BOATING EQUIPMENT

In emergency situations where the proper equipment is not available, it is necessary to improvise. A shirt or a coat can be made into a sling for a broken arm. Old sails are useful in numerous ways. Pieces of board, mop handles wrapped in cloth, etc., can be used as splints. A blanket can be made into a stretcher by taking several turns of the material around an oar on each side. A pail containing sand or water will serve as a weight for the suspension of a dislocated shoulder. There are dozens of ways in which one may provide clever, effective first-aid substitutes by using on-the-spot materials and the imagination. See page 93–95 for illustrations of typical improvisations.

In the field on a dive, one can never carry all the first-aid equipment one might like. However, the equipment you dive with has many uses in first aid. Here is a list—and you will probably think of many more uses.

MASK

Mask as a bandage for head or eye wound.
Mask as a cup.

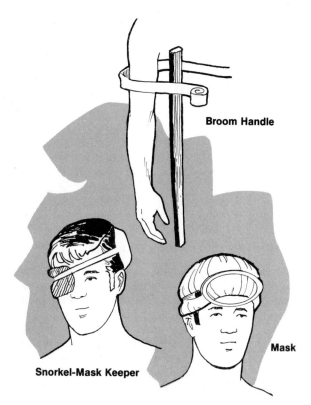

Broom Handle

Mask

Snorkel-Mask Keeper

USE OF "ON-THE-SPOT" EQUIPMENT FOR FIRST AID

Straps can be used for a tourniquet.
Straps can be used for bandaging.

SNORKEL

Airway if mouth is too damaged for mouth-to-mouth re-
    suscitation.
Tourniquet bar.

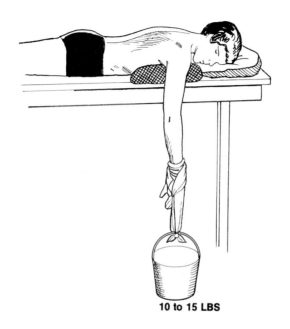

10 to 15 LBS

REDUCTION OF A DISLOCATED SHOULDER

Splint for finger. If so used, split side of snorkel first to
  allow for swelling.
Snorkel to mask keeper can be used as a small bandage.

FINS

Back brace for small child.
Splint.
Neck brace to immobilize head and neck.
Fan for heatstroke or heat exhaustion.
Tourniquet may be made with heel strap and fin buckle.

WET SUIT

Insulation for shock victims.
Pillow.
Pressure bandage.
Padding for splints.
Dressing.
Bandages or tourniquet strap if cut into strips.
Improvised stretcher by running poles through arms and
    legs.
Arm sling.

BUOYANCY COMPENSATOR

Carrying water.
Material can be used for dressing.
Waist strap, crotch strap, hose can serve as tourniquet
    strap.
Partially inflated BC may serve as an inflatable splint.
CO_2 cartridges might be used as a finger splint.
Can be used in making an arm sling.
Pillow.

KNIFE

General cutting.
Splint (sheath).
Straps for tourniquet or bandages.
Knife as a tourniquet bar.
Pressure bandage.

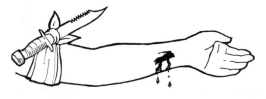

USE OF KNIFE FOR TOURNIQUET BAR

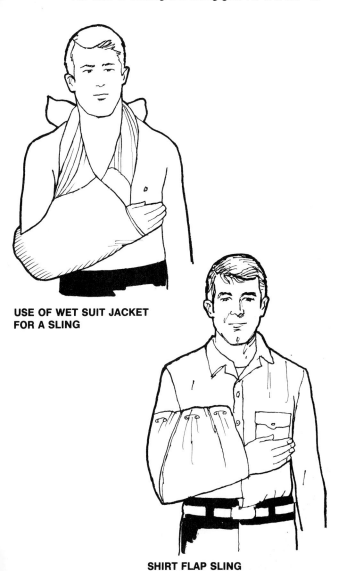

**USE OF WET SUIT JACKET
FOR A SLING**

SHIRT FLAP SLING

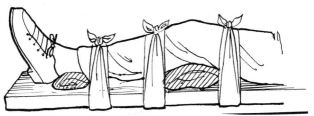

SPLINTING FRACTURED KNEECAP

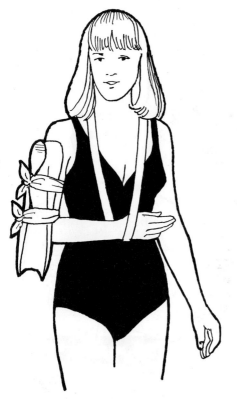

USE OF FIN AS SPLINT AND TANK STRAP AS SLING

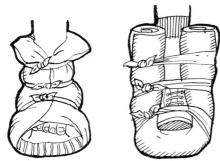

IMPROVISED SPLINTS WITH PILLOW AND BLANKET

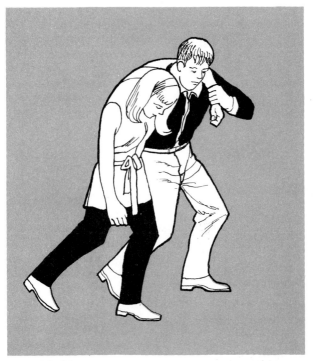

ASSIST CARRY

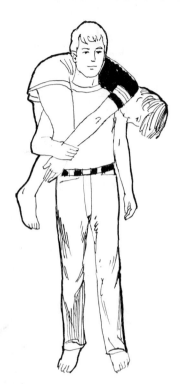

FIREMAN'S CARRY

GAME BAG

Arm sling.
Some types can be used as bandages.
Some can be used as dressing.
Metal frame opening of bag may serve as a splint.
Padding for splints.

SPEARS

Poles for stretcher bars.
Supports for shade tents.
Splints.
Line for bandages.
Crutch or cane.

5
First-aid kit for divers

The first-aid kit should be a sound, well-made box of durable, moistureproof construction. Appropriate first-aid materials should be part of any dive preparation. The following articles should be included:

1. Box of adhesive compresses (assorted sizes).
2. Package of 3″ x 3″ sterile gauze pads individually packed.
3. 2″ roller bandages.
4. Large gauze dressings 12″ x 12″, sterile.
5. Two or three triangular bandages.
6. Pair of scissors.
7. Pair of tweezers.
8. Dowel ½″ x 6″ for tourniquets.
9. Plastic box of baking soda.
10. Box of aspirin (5-gram tablets).
11. Antihistamine tablets and ointment. (These should be available without prescription.)
12. Meat tenderizer with papaya extract dissolved in water for local application; helpful in reducing the effects of jellyfish and Portuguese Man-of-War stings.
13. Package of Band-Aids.
14. Bottle of iodine or mercurochrome, or tincture of zephiran (benzalkonium chloride), a good marine antiseptic.

15. Roll of adhesive tape.
16. Pack of single-edge razor blades.
17. Clean needle.
18. Chapstick.
19. Small bottle of fresh water.
20. Motion-sickness pills.
21. Thermometer.

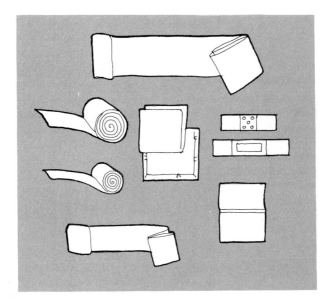

TYPES OF BANDAGES

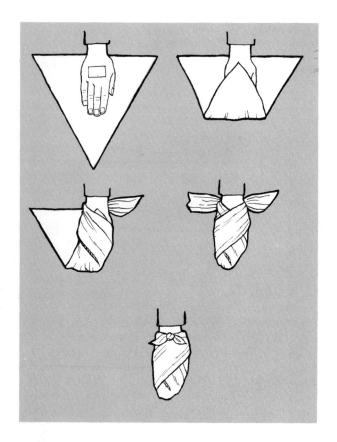

TRIANGULAR HAND BANDAGE

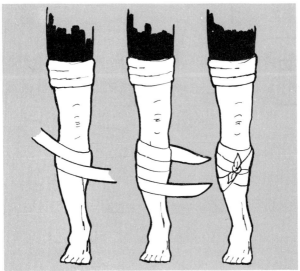

LEG BANDAGE

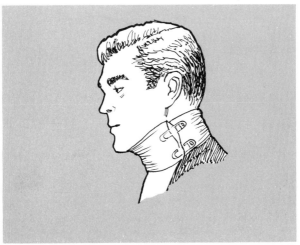

NECK BANDAGE

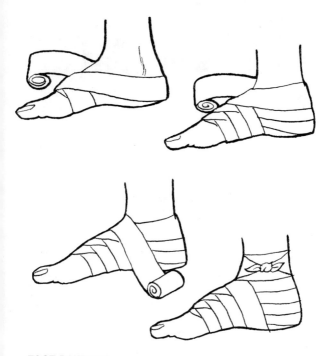

FOOT BANDAGE

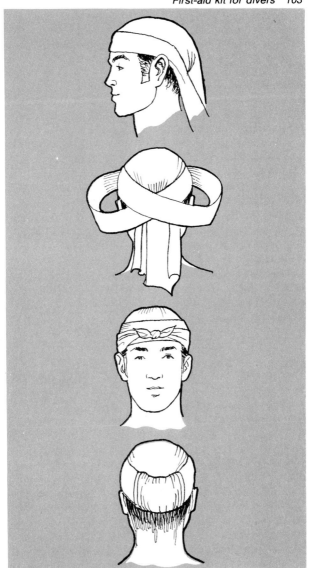

TRIANGULAR HEAD BANDAGE

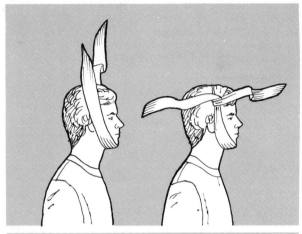

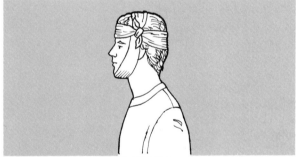

BANDAGE FOR A JAW FRACTURE

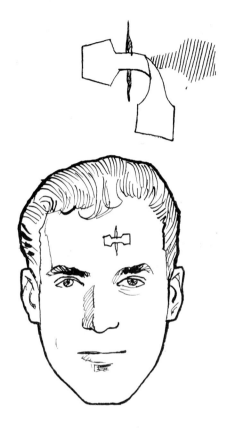

APPLYING A BUTTERFLY STRIP

6
First-aid kit for boaters

1. Four large triangular bandages. These are for slings, regular bandages or pads when folded. They can be used to cover large areas. They come prepacked clean but not sterile.
2. Nonadhesive sterile dressings, 3" x 3" or 4" x 4". Carry one dozen. These are prepacked and sterile.
3. Elastoplast adhesive bandage. Carry one 3" and one 4". They are used to strap up sprains and fasten dressings to any portion of the body.
4. Twelve yards of surgical gauze. This can be used to make up pads as well as serving as bandages.
5. An eye pad. If you don't have one, use nonadherent sterile dressing to make one.
6. Assorted adhesive wound dressings for minor cuts.
7. Antihistamine cream. Can be used for bites, stings and minor burns.
8. Paracetamol tablets, 500 mg per tablet. Used for the relief of pain. For children use paracetamol elixir, 120 mg per 5 ml for pain.
9. Motion-sickness pills. See your pharmacist.
10. If you plan to be away for a while, carry antibiotics. You will need to get a prescription from a doctor to

buy these. Suggest tetracycline in 250-mg tablets. This is a broad-spectrum antibiotic.

11. Scissors.
12. Tweezers.
13. Sodium chloride tablets for heat cramps.
14. Insect repellent.
15. Thermometer, clinical.
16. Sunscreen lotion for protection against sunburn.

DIVER FIRST-AID COMMANDMENTS

1. First-aid training helps avoid panic.
2. Think and identify the problem and first aid required.
3. Act calmly, quickly, effectively.
4. Note the circumstances of the accident for the doctor's use.
5. Know your sources of help in advance.
6. In advance, list closest recompression chambers by address and telephone number.
7. Carry a first-aid kit in your diving gear and this booklet as a handy reference.
8. Drill and review first aid with your dive buddies.
9. Log and report all accidents.
10. Know your subject—*First Aid.*

ABOUT THE COUNCIL FOR NATIONAL COOPERATION IN AQUATICS (CNCA)

The Council for National Cooperation in Aquatics was founded in 1951. It is comprised of 33 national organizations, each with a specific interest in aquatics. The member organizations are noncommercial. CNCA is an educational, nongovernmental, public-service organization whose member groups come together annually to discuss problems of mutual concern and to work collectively for solutions to common problems.

This collaborative effort has had broad and useful results for the whole field of aquatic endeavor, ranging from scuba training to swimming-pool design and lifeguard training, from water programming to swimming for the handicapped, as well as methods for improving the quality of life for urban dwellers.

The Council's concern for the care and safety of participants in aquatic activities finds expression in products made available to the member organizations and from them to the public in the form of improved aquatic program design. CNCA keeps in touch with international aquatic developments and is well represented abroad. This international exchange further enriches the world aquatic picture.

CONSTITUENT GROUPS

National Organizations That Constitute CNCA
Amateur Athletic Union of the U.S. (AAU)
American Academy of Pediatrics (AAP)
American Alliance for Health, Physical Education &
   Recreation (AAHPER)
   —General Representation (AAHPER-Staff)
   —Aquatic Council of AAHPER
American Camping Association (ACA)
American National Red Cross (ARC)
American Public Health Association (APHA)
American Swimming Coaches Association (ASCA)
Athletic Institute (AI)
Boy Scouts of America (BSA)
Boys' Clubs of America (BCA)
Camp Fire Girls, Inc. (CFG)
Girl Scouts of America (GSA)
Joseph P. Kennedy Jr. Foundation (JPKJF)
National Aquatic Forum (NAF)
National Association of Intercollegiate Athletics (NAIA)
National Association of Underwater Instructors (NAUI)
National Board of the Young Women's Christian
   Association (YWCA)
National Collegiate Athletic Association (NCAA)

National Council of Young Men's Christian Association
(YMCA)
  —General Representation (YMCA-Staff)
  —National YMCA Operating Council on Aquatics
  (NYOCA)
National Federation of State High School Athletic
Associations (NFSHSAA)
National Forum for Advancement of Aquatics (NFAA)
National Industrial Recreation Association (NIRA)
National Jewish Welfare Board (JWB)
National Jr. College Athletic Association (NJCAA)
National Recreation & Park Association (NRPA)
National Safety Council (NSC)
National Swimming Pool Institute (NSPI)
President's Council on Physical Fitness & Sports
(PCPFS)
Professional Association of Diving Instructors (P.A.D.I.)
Underwater Society of America (USA)
United States Office of Education (USOE)
United States Life Saving Association (USLA)

National Organizations That Constitute CCCA
Allied Boating Federation (ABF)
Boy Scouts of Canada (BSC)
Boys' Clubs of Canada (BCC)
Canadian Amateur Diving Association (CADA)
Canadian Amateur Swimming Association (CASA)
Canadian Amateur Synchronized Swimming Association
(CASSA)
Canadian Armed Forces (CAF)
Canadian Association for Health, Physical Education &
Recreation (CAHPER)
Canadian Camping Association (CCA)
Canadian Intercollegiate Athletic Union (CIAU)
Canadian Parks & Recreation Association (CPRA)
Canadian Power Squadrons (CPS)
Canadian Recreational Canoeing Association (CRCA)
Canadian White Water Association (CWWA)

Canadian Red Cross Society (CRCS)
Canadian Safety Council (CSC)
Canadian Swimming Pool Federation (CSPF)
Association of Canadian Underwater Councils (ACUC)
Canadian Water Polo Association (CWPA)
Canadian Water Ski Association (CWSA)
Canadian Yachting Association (CYA)
Girl Guides of Canada (GGC)
Ministry of Transport (MOT)
National Association of Underwater Instructors of
   Canada (NAUIC)
National Council of Young Men's Christian Association
   of Canada (YMCA)
Naval Officers' Association of Canada (NOAC)
Royal Life Saving Society of Canada (RLSSC)
Sports Federation of Canada (SFC)
Sport Participation Canada (SPC)
Young Men's Hebrew Association (YMHA)
Young Women's Christian Association of Canada
   (YMCA)

SEA GRANT

The National Sea Grant Program is concerned with the development and wise use of the ocean's resources. It was established in 1966 to accelerate research, education, and advisory services in marine resources, including their conservation, proper management, and social and economic utilization. The term "Sea Grant" was chosen to emphasize its parallel with the century-old "Land Grant" program. The term is used to point out how the present needs of the nation in the marine environment compare with the needs for developing the nation's agricultural lands in the 1860s. The Sea Grant Program follows the pattern of the Land Grant by providing the means through which scholars, institutions of higher learning and others can apply their knowledge and talents to the practical needs of the nation and the world. It

includes the Land Grant concept of advisory and extension services which have marine advisory agents located
throughout the coastal and Great Lakes regions to assist
commercial and recreational fishermen, seafood proces-
sors, and others with their marine problems and to speed
up the introduction of the latest results of scientific research in the marine educational, scientific, commercial
and recreational communities. The Office of Sea Grant,
National Oceanic and Atmospheric Administration
(NOAA), administers the National Sea Grant Program.
Through a matching fund program, that office provides
financial grants-in-aid to colleges and universities and to
other groups and individuals carrying out research and
educational projects in marine resources.

Index

alcohol, use of, 88
appendicitis, 41
artificial circulation (external cardiac compression), 24
artificial respiration. *See* mouth-to-mouth resuscitation
asphyxia. *See* stoppage of breathing

bites. *See* stings and bites
bleeding, 8
  arterial pressure points, 10
  tourniquet, 10
  underwater, 9
boating and diving gear, use for first aid, 89
boating equipment, emergency use of, 85
broken back, 29
broken bones, 28
broken neck, 29
burns, 32
  chemical, 36
  electrical, 36
  extent of (rule of nines), 37, 38

carbon-dioxide excess (hypercapnia), 85
carbon-monoxide poisoning, 85
cardiopulmonary resuscitation (CPR), 23
childbirth, 66
chilling/hypothermia, 51

choking, 19
cold, exposure to, 53, 55
colds, 63

decompression sickness, 78
dermatitis, 57
dislocated joints, 31
diver first-aid commandments, 107
diving above sea level, 87
drowning, 16, 86

ear
  external ear infection, 39
  middle ear infection, 60
  wax: impacted, 58
earache, 59
electric shock, 38
embolism, air, 79
emphysema. *See* mediastinal emphysema *and* subcutaneous emphysema
exhaustion syndrome, 56

fainting, 38
first-aid kit
  for boaters, 106
  for divers, 98
flying after diving, 88
frostbite, 53, 55

head injury, 31
heart attack, 22
heart failure, 23
heatstroke, 56

Heimlich Maneuver, 20
hernia. *See* rupture
hypercapnia. *See* carbon-
    dioxide excess
hyperventilation, 82
hypothermia. *See*
    chilling/hypothermia
hypoxia. *See* oxygen shortage

injuries caused by marine life,
    69–77

marijuana, use of, 88
mediastinal emphysema, 80
motion sickness, 57
mouth-to-mouth resuscitation,
    17
moving the injured, 32

nitrogen narcosis, 85
nosebleed, 43

oxygen shortage (hypoxia), 83
oxygen toxicity, 84

pneumothorax, 81
poisoning
    antidote, 41
    carbon monoxide, 85
    contact by eyes or skin, 40
    by inhaling, 41
    by mouth 39
    from plants, 41
    by swallowing, 40

rule of nines, 37, 38
rupture (hernia), 63

sea sickness. *See* motion
    sickness
shock, 12

sinusitis, 62
snakebites, 47
sore throat, 61
splints, 25
sprains, 42
squeeze, 82
    lung, 83
    mask, 83
    sinus, 82
stings and bites, 44. *See also*
    snakebites
    animal, 51
    black widow, 46
    brown recluse, 46
    human, 51
    scorpion, 45
    spider, 46
    tarantula, 46
stoppage of breathing
    (asphyxia), 16
strains, 42
strangulation, 19
stroke, 64
subcutaneous emphysema, 81

tetanus, 28
toothache, 65

unconscious diver, 82

vomiting, 38

wound care, 26

Association Press
Follett Publishing Company/Chicago

ISBN 0-695-8 **1425**-7